Understanding and cop[...]

THE
FACTS
ABOUT
CANCER

Causes, Cures, Treatment, Prevention

Ian J. Forbes

OXFORD UNIVERSITY PRESS AUSTRALIA

Oxford New York Toronto
Delhi Bombay Calcutta Madras Karachi
Petaling Jaya Singapore Hong Kong Tokyo
Nairobi Dar es Salaam Cape Town
Melbourne Auckland
and associated companies in Berlin Ibadan

OXFORD is a trade mark of Oxford University Press

National Library of Australia
Cataloguing-in-Publication data:
  Forbes, Ian J. (Ian James), 1930-
    The facts about cancer.

    Bibliography.
    ISBN 0 19 553188 4.

    1. Cancer - Dictionaries. 2. Cancer - Popular works.
    I. Title.

    616.994003

Designed by Peter Shaw
Typeset by Best-set Typesetter Ltd., Hong Kong
Printed in Australia by The Book Printer, Victoria
Published by Oxford University Press,
253 Normanby Road, South Melbourne, Australia

Introduction

From a historical perspective ... the rate (of progress) has accelerated so rapidly in the past 40 years that it is reasonable to believe that the avoidable causes of all the principal cancers will soon be discovered and that it will not be long before we can reduce the risk of developing serious forms of the disease from one in three or four, as it is now, to less than one in ten.

Sir Richard Doll, 1988

Who needs to know about cancer? This may be answered by describing a case.

In 1978 a 25-year-old woman, Mrs M, mother of two children, noticed a lump in her neck when she was showering. As it was painless, she forgot about it for a few days.

Fortunately for herself, her husband and the two children, she mentioned the lump to a friend, a former nurse, who advised an immediate appointment with her doctor. The lump was removed under general anaesthetic at the earliest opportunity.

Within a few days Mrs M was informed that she had *Hodgkin's disease.

Consider Mrs M's needs and the needs of her family. She did not know what Hodgkin's disease was, she did not understand exactly what cancer was and she knew nothing of what she would have to go through.

She knew fear. She needed some certainties. Her husband knew no more than she.

Mrs M, like every other person who is given the diagnosis of cancer, immediately wanted answers to questions that had suddenly become vital. What would she have to go through? What does *radiotherapy do? What is *chemotherapy? How did she get this cancer? Was it due to something in the *environment? Was her *occupation to blame? Was her *lifestyle or her *diet at fault? Was is her *heredity? Could a *virus have caused it?

Her husband and members of her family also needed to know.

With the passage of time Mrs M and her husband came to appreciate the sophisticated medical services of a Western civilization. Also for the first time they fully appreciated the benefits of medical research, for Hodgkin's disease is a cancer that has become curable only in the past twenty years, as a direct result of painstaking studies.

Mrs M also learnt that some people were ignorant of things she believed they should know. A friend in the **local municipal council** knew little about the cancer risks associated with toxic *chemical wastes and she came to realise that waste disposal in her district ignored some of these risks. A **factory manager** seemed to know little about the cancer hazards of his industry. She learnt more than her **local doctor** could tell her about *diet and cancer and where to get help for some of her needs. She did not get answers to her questions from some of her **nurses** or from the local **pharmacist**. Her local **member of parliament** did not seem to know much about cancer or to be keen to support cancer research.

Mrs M's story ended happily. After medical examinations and laboratory tests, she underwent prescribed courses of radiotherapy and chemotherapy. Now, ten years later, she does not need further annual checks, because the risk of recurrence has passed.

This story is intended to illustrate why information about cancer is needed by people in all walks of life. Cancer is a big problem and it is increasing as our population ages, but we should not, through ignorance, deny ourselves the chance of beating it. The only way to combat cancer is through knowledge. Knowledge also helps conquer fear. Through knowledge, **the majority of cancers can be avoided or dealt with early enough for a cure to be effected.**

Sooner or later, cancer affects almost everybody in one way or another, either personally, or as a member of a victim's family, or as a friend of a victim. Lives are affected, sometimes irrevocably, when cancer strikes mothers, breadwinners and leaders in the community.

We would all like a society free from cancer, but understanding by scientists is not enough. Not all of the available knowledge is being put to good use, because the level of understanding in the community is too low. Simply by applying the knowledge that is already available, countless humans could be spared the miseries of cancer.

Defeating cancer is the responsibility of the whole of society. **Everybody** has a responsibility for his or her own health. **Every family** must have informed views about *diet and *lifestyle. Every citizen should know about *prevention, *screening facilities, and *warning signs of cancer.

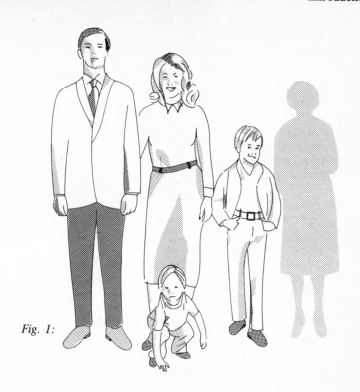

Fig. 1:

Cancer affects almost everybody, sooner or later

Governments must make courageous decisions to ensure a cancer-safe environment and must ensure that facilities for treatment match the possibilities. However, governments can only introduce measures to fight cancer when public opinion is sufficiently persuasive. The quality of governmental decisions depends upon the enlightenment of the community. *Asbestos was used long after its cancer-inducing properties were known. Only when the public was informed and opinion was strong enough was it possible for governments to prevail against entrenched interests.

The aim of this book is to make essential knowledge about cancer available and understandable to those who need it, that is, not only to people in paramedical professions, in positions of responsibility in industry and government, and to cancer patients themselves, but to all of us.

Using This Book

This book is intended to meet several requirements. Some will want to refer to it from time to time for information about a single topic, such as the safety or danger of a chemical substance, so that a decision can be made.

Others will have the need to know what the implications of a certain cancer or a particular treatment are.

Some will urgently need help in coping with cancer. Many want to understand what cancer is.

To fulfil these requirements, the book has been structured in dictionary form. A word preceded by a star (*) has its own entry. For example, in the entry **gene** are found *genetic code, *protein and *chromosome, each having its own entry, usually containing a definition and more information.

It is suggested that those who want to use the book as a text should read the major essays first, then the various leads may be followed up.

A

ABMT autologous bone marrow transplanation. See *bone marrow transplantation.

acoustic neuroma also known as eighth cranial nerve tumour, a *benign tumour that grows on the nerve for hearing, which is curable if it has not grown too large or if *surgery is not too difficult. Acoustic neuroma causes deafness, ringing in the involved ear, and in the advanced stages headaches and loss of balance. See *brain cancer.

acrylonitrile chemical used in the plastics industry, suspected of causing cancer. See *occupation and cancer.

acyclovir medication used to treat *shingles (herpes zoster). To be effective treatment must begin early, preferably before the rash has developed. Acyclovir may cause side effects on the *bone marrow, similar to those caused by many agents used in cancer chemotherapy, leading to a reduction of red and white blood cells and *platelets in the circulation. Acyclovir is administered by intravenous injection over several days.

addiction physical or emotional dependence on a drug, associated with compulsion to obtain and use it. True addicts have a strong tendency to relapse into their former state of addiction after withdrawal of the drug. Many patients are concerned about addiction if they take *morphine or other addictive drugs for relief of severe pain. They fear that control of their lives will be lost. However, patients who use narcotics for control of pain usually do not become addicted as do persons who use narcotics for emotional and social reasons, and they can usually stop using them if pain can be controlled by other treatment.
   In the great majority of cases, proper use of major pain-relieving drugs restores value to the lives of patients who are crippled by pain. See *treatment, *pain.

adjuvant chemotherapy *chemotherapy after surgery for *breast and other cancers intended to reduce the rate of 'recurrence' of the cancer. 'Recurrence' is actually the growth of cancer seedlings that had spread from the primary site before the time of operation.

Adriamycin trade name for doxorubicin, drug used in *chemotherapy

adult T cell leukaemia cancer of blood cells found mainly in Southern Japan, in the Caribbean islands and in many parts of Africa. The cancer is caused by a recently-discovered virus, *human T leukaemia virus type I (HTLV-I). See *leukaemia, *lymphoma.

HTLV-I virus spreads among members of families, particularly from parents to children. The incubation period of the cancer is many years, perhaps 20 or more. Adult T cell leukaemia is found occasionally in non-endemic areas.

It is of great interest that this virus is closely related to the *human immunodeficiency virus (HIV), which causes *AIDS. These human viruses may have evolved from very similar viruses in African monkeys.

aflatoxin a poison in foodstuffs affected by the mould *Aspergillus flavus*, which causes cancer of the *liver, principally in Southern Africa. Aflatoxin came to notice when 100,000 turkeys died in England from acute liver destruction. The trouble was traced to peanut meal infected with the *Aspergillus* mould. Aflatoxin was then shown to cause liver cancers in rats. Aflatoxin probably acts together with *hepatitis B virus (HBV) to cause liver cancer in Africa.

ageing and cancer *Epidemiological studies confirm that cancer is linked with age. In Western countries life expectancy has increased as much as 30% in the past 35 years, largely as a result of reducing diseases of the heart and circulation. During this time the cancer death rate for men has increased 30–40%. Until recently there has been no increase for women.

The figures tell us that the risk of cancer increases with age, but they do not tell us whether this increase in cancer is inevitable or not. Either cancer may develop because of an unavoidable tendency in ourselves, associated with our makeup, or because we fall victim to something in our environment.

There was a common belief that cancer would occur with ageing, whatever precautions were taken; external factors were thought merely to influence which types of cancer occurred, not how many. We now know that this is not true. All the evidence indicates that the increased incidence of cancer that has occurred in the older people during this century is due to a change in the world, not in the people. While the percentage of the American population over 60 years of age doubled from 7% in 1900 to 14% in 1960, the incidence of cancer in people over 60 more than doubled. In other words, the risk of cancer in older people is greater now than it was at the beginning of the century.

Calculations indicate that the increase, over and above that due to age, is about 0.55% per annum. This increase is due to factors in the *environment or *lifestyle. Some studies suggest that the recent increase is almost all due to the increase of *lung cancer in women. See also *air pollution, *water.

Agent Orange US military code name for a mixture of herbicides
*2,4-D and *2,4,5-T used as a defoliant during 1965–70 in the war
in Vietnam. Agent Orange was unintentionally contaminated with
*dioxin.

AIDS acquired immunodeficiency syndrome, caused by the *human
immunodeficiency virus (HIV), which exerts its deadly effects by
killing particular members of the body's white blood cell defence
force. Unchecked infection by a number of other viruses is thought to
cause cancers in AIDS sufferers.
   Cancers occur in the *tongue, lower end of *bowel and *skin.
*Lymphomas also occur. Before the AIDS epidemic, a *skin cancer
called *Kaposi's sarcoma was rarely seen except in tropical Africa and
amongst Mediterranean Jews. Kaposi's sarcoma in AIDS patients
appears to develop in response to unchecked infection with a common and normally mild virus, the *cytomegalovirus. Chronic myeloid
*leukaemia, which usually occurs in middle-aged and elderly people,
also occurs in patients with AIDS.

air pollution The pollutants in outdoor and indoor air are similar.
Indoor pollutants may reach high levels because they are emitted into
a small volume, from which they cannot escape readily. Many air
pollutants are considered to be capable of increasing the likelihood of
cancer developing. Heating appliances that burn natural gas,
kerosene, oil and wood all release varying proportions of *benzpyrene, *nitrogen oxides, *methylene chloride, *formaldehyde and
trace organic chemicals. *Nitrosamines can be produced from oxides
of nitrogen. Sulphur dioxide causes acid haze which blocks out the
wavelength of light that induces the skin to form *vitamin D. See
*ultraviolet light.
   One of the most important indoor pollutants is *tobacco smoke.
Other indoor pollutants include chemicals that are given off by building materials, cleaning fluids (including *benzene), *organochlorine
pesticides, paint and *radon. *Asbestos particles can be released from
insulating materials in older buildings. The house dust mite, fungi and
bacteria are also indoor pollutants that do not seem to have a bearing
on cancer.
   Incineration of municipal and industrial wastes processes these
materials, but does not dispose of them entirely, because some of the
waste pollutes the atmosphere. Apart from organochlorines, *dioxins
and oxides of nitrogen and sulphur, *metals are dispersed into the
atmosphere by incineration of waste and by metal *foundries.
   Air pollution in houses and buildings depends greatly on ventilation. Houses which are in warm climates and are open to breezes
have less polluted air than large buildings, particularly in cold climates, because of measures in the latter to reduce energy loss. Poor

quality indoor air in large modern buildings has been blamed for the *sick office syndrome, which has been the subject of recent attention by the media.

Estimates of the cancer risks of indoor pollution put inhalation of benzene, benzepyrene, other *polycylic hydrocarbons and other inhaled carcinogens equal to the risk of *passive smoking and one 30,000th of the risk of cigarette smoking. Indoor *radon can range from being as dangerous as cigarette smoking in some houses, to being 60 times less dangerous, that is, equal to the chance we all have of dying from a household accident.

Expert opinion attributes 7% of cancers to environmental and occupational pollution. Pollution contributes mainly to *lung cancer. It has been estimated that about 30 lung cancers arise from air pollution in the Sydney region each year. Air pollution in Japan adds to lung cancers in industrial areas, particularly along the coast, where the air pollution is worst. Passive smoking increases the rates of lung and *cervix cancers in wives of smokers. See *chemicals as causes of cancer.

alcohol   From time immemorial alcohol has been both a solace and a scourge for mankind. We now dignify it with the classification of recreational drug. It must come as a relief to many to know that among all the things we like and should not indulge ourselves in, alcohol is not too bad as a cancer risk factor. To those who suffer from having to give up *tobacco, there is some consolation in knowing that as far as the risk of cancer goes, alcohol is not one of the major culprits. Neither, however, can it be completely exonerated. It has been estimated that avoidance of alcohol would prevent 3% of cancers.

Alcohol, particularly in the form of spirits and together with tobacco, is a factor in development of cancer of the *tongue, mouth and *oesophagus (gullet). It is a factor in causing primary cancer of the *liver, a rare condition in Australian society, but a risk for alcoholics who suffer gross damage to the liver.

Alcohol is now considered to increase the risk of *breast cancer slightly, i.e. by a factor of 1·3. See *lifestyle and cancer.

aldrin   *chlorinated insecticide. See *chemicals as causes of cancer.

alopecia   loss of hair. See *chemotherapy, side effects of.

alternative cancer treatments   The term *alternative treatment* is used to embrace all treatments which are not accepted as orthodox by the medical profession. The difference is based on proof of effectiveness. Every orthodox treatment has to undergo testing and is described precisely in textbooks or journals. Alternative treatments are not described precisely in any available reference texts.

Orthodox treatments are based on scientific studies, reports of which are available to everybody through national and international systems of information exchange. The types of tests they have undergone and the results of the tests are all available in the medical and scientific literature.

Some recoveries from cancer will occur, whatever treatment is being given at the time. Those using alternative treatments may attribute such recoveries to these treatments, without recognizing that they have occurred by chance, that is, through factors unrelated to the treatment. Before any cancer remedy can responsibly be offered to the public it must be tested in large numbers of patients.

What appear to be miraculous cures may also occur in patients misdiagnosed as having cancer. Usually the diagnosis in these cases has not been confirmed by *biopsy.

Orthodox medical treatments are effective in only a proportion of cancer patients, but the frequency of such responses has been documented, while no such information is available for alternative treatments.

Every scientist or medical practitioner who believes he or she can contribute an advance in the treatment of cancer, or indeed any other disease, has to provide the evidence that his or her contribution is truly an advance. This proof involves a proper *clinical trial, a strict comparison of treatments, which shows that a new treatment B produces more benefit than the best currently available treatment A. This can only be concluded if proper criteria of benefit were chosen before the trial, if the difference is statistically significant, and if adequate precautions were taken to rule out other factors that could be influencing the result. Then the side-effects must be evaluated to show that the disadvantages of the new treatment are not too serious.

There are many pitfalls in evaluating new treatments. One of these is the *placebo effect. Any medication given with confidence and assurance may be scored as effective for a while, because of the power of suggestion and the desire of the patient to believe in a good effect.

Almost every patient with cancer has to face perplexing questions and advice about cancer treatments offered by people who do not belong to the medical profession. Most patients will be caused anguish by well-meaning friends who insist that they know of a cure for the very cancer they are suffering from, although the medical profession cannot cure them.

Alternative treatments offer hope when the medical profession cannot give it. Alternative treatments may also give the patient a sense of control over his or her own destiny, a feeling of contributing to his or her own individual case. It is easy for a patient to feel that the doctor is looking at him or her in a statistical sense, as a number rather than a person.

Alternative cancer treatments

Alternative cancer treatments are flourishing. American patients are said to spend $4 billion annually on alternative treatments, ranging from outright frauds to methods which are, at best, questionable.

A substance known as *laetrile, amygdalin or krebiozen is perhaps the most notorious of the alternative remedies. It was written in 1984 that 'the nation (USA) appears to have weathered the laetrile phenomenon ... just having passed through the greatest episode of quackery in our history' (quoted from Lerner, see References in Appendix). The more the medical profession condemned the substance, the greater the public outcry at the apparent wrong perpetrated against it. What is referred to as the 'laetrile phenomenon' has been analysed extensively to find reasons why the public wanted to ignore scientific evidence. In fact, many properly conducted studies failed to find any anti-cancer effect of laetrile. However, many seek something more reassuring than plain medical explanation with acknowledgement of limitations.

The most popular alternative treatments today are '*metabolic therapy' and 'diet therapy'.

The most common of the diet therapies is the so-called 'macrobiotic diet'. The prescribed regime is usually rather unpleasant and tedious to produce. Wheat grass features in versions of the macrobiotic diet.

Other alternative treatments include the use of *vitamins, *retinoic acid and various forms of so-called *immunotherapy.

Patients should discuss with their doctors alternative therapies that have been suggested to them. There is no reason why patients should be refused any reasonable discussion and explanation of matters that vitally concern them. If responses to their questions are not satisfactory, patients are urged most strongly to obtain opinions from other independent specialists.

Doctors who care for cancer patients are very much aware of alternative therapies. No doctor who values his or her reputation would refuse any treatment that may be helpful to a patient. In many cases, unorthodox treatments do no harm and can be given together with the orthodox. It is always possible that there is something new in an alternative treatment and a good doctor will not deny the possibility of benefit from a treatment about which he or she has no expert knowledge.

Doctors are bound to point out the disadvantages of alternative therapies. One is the disillusionment that follows when they fail. It is tragic when patients who stand a good chance of benefit from orthodox treatment reject this chance in favour of a treatment that offers little.

Unfortunately, many alternative therapies offer hope in the short term, but patients who refuse orthodox treatment which offers a good chance of cure are usually betrayed in the long term, often at great cost in money, and to their great anguish.

A question of great importance is: does the attitude of the cancer patient affect the course of his or her disease? There are reputable studies of patients that demonstrate improvements in mood, adjustment to their condition and help with pain, from group therapy, psychological help and social support. Some patients obtain strength and peace of mind from *meditation. However, there are few studies of the effect of psychological help on survival. This was the subject of a recent *clinical trial, involving 86 women who had incurable breast cancer, which was published recently in the 'Lancet' (see references to Spiegel and Lancet in the Appendix). Fifty of these women were given psychological and social help and met for 90 minutes every week for a year in small groups together with a therapist, whose breast cancer had responded to treatment (although it was probably not cured). This group was compared with a control group of 36 women whose disease and medical treatment were similar, but who did not receive psychological and social help. Those who received the psychosocial treatment survived 18 months longer than the control group.

The 'Lancet' encouraged its readers in sober terms 'to adopt the same healthy scepticism about these claims as they would about the claims of any other breakthrough in the therapy of metastatic cancer', but ended its comments with the concession that the measures which were used were 'at least life-enhancing, in stark contrast to the life impoverishment suffered by many terminally ill patients subjected to the vile diets, costly *placebos and exhausting introspections recommended by the more lunatic fringe among alternative practitioners'.

anaemia   deficiency of red blood cells in the blood. This can arise in cancer from bleeding, for example, into the bowel or from failure to make enough red cells. See *bowel cancer, *stomach cancer.

aluminium sulphate   chemical added to *water, not known to cause cancer, but a possible cause of Alzheimer's dementia.

Ames test   a test to show the potential of chemical substances to cause *mutations—damage to *DNA—in bacteria. Cancer results from damage to DNA. A positive result in the Ames test is therefore an indication that a chemical may cause cancer, but does not prove that it is a powerful cause of cancer in humans, because many factors influence the induction of cancer. For example, a substance that is positive in the Ames test may affect different animal species quite differently. See *causes of cancer.

amino acid   building block of *protein. Amino acids, of which there are 20, are used by all living matter to make protein. Amino acids are made by *enzymes from smaller molecules. There are specific words in the *genetic code for each amino acid. All living matter draws upon the same pool of amino acids to make protein and the codewords are the same for each species.

aminoglutethimide medication used in treatment of *breast cancer. Aminoglutethimide acts by blocking production of sex *hormones in the adrenal glands and also blocks *cortisone production. Persons taking aminoglutethimide must always take regular cortisone to meet the body's requirements. See *chemotherapy.

4-aminobiphenyl carcinogenic chemical of the *aromatic amine class. See *chemicals as causes of cancer, *occupation and cancer.

amosite brown *asbestos.

androgen general name for male sex hormones, which determine male characteristics such as growth of facial hair.

aniline dyes and aromatic amines Factories to manufacture a new class of dye were founded in Europe in the last half of the 19th century. Aniline was a starting point for the new dyes and the methods of production provided every opportunity for workers to inhale fumes and to touch the compounds. The crystals were even sorted by hand. *Bladder cancer was eventually related to the new occupations associated with aniline dye manufacture.

The principal *carcinogen from aniline dye manufacture is the derivative beta-*naphthylamine. *Bladder cancer appeared in workers who had stopped working in dye factories for as long as 35 years. The long lead time before the cancer was detected made it hard to recognize the connection between the chemical and the cancer. Anoher derivative of aniline, butter yellow (dimethyl-aminoazobenzene, DAB) was added to margarine until it was proved to be a carcinogen.

Many of the aniline dyes are in the chemical class known as *aromatic amines, which includes *naphthylamine, *4-amino-biphenyl, *4-nitrophenyl and *ortho-toluidine. These substances are all strongly suspected to cause bladder cancer and are present in *tobacco smoke. See *chemicals as causes of cancer, *occupation and cancer.

angiogenesis factor *growth factor that stimulates growth of blood vessels in normal tissues and tumours. See *nature of cancer.

ankylosing spondylitis type of arthritis mainly affecting the spine. Previously, treatment of this condition by *X-rays caused the development of *multiple myeloma, a tumour of the *bone marrow which destroys bone. See *bone cancer.

Anti-cancer Societies, Foundations, or Cancer Councils, organizations in most English-speaking countries for support of research into cancer and support for cancer patients. See *coping with cancer, *help for cancer patients. Addresses of the various Austrialian Anti-Cancer Societies are listed in the Appendix.

antibody substance made by the body to neutralize infections. Because of their matching shape, antibodies blanket part of the surface of the invading microorganism. Antibodies are *proteins that can be separated from the blood by chemical procedures, into the *gamma globulin fraction. Gamma globulin is readily available for patients whose immune defences are weakened by chemotherapy, cancer or other disease and offers protection against the common infections, particularly those affecting the lungs. It is given monthly or more frequently, by injection.
   *Monoclonal antibodies, made by cells in the laboratory, can be designed as a treatment to attack cancers. See *immunity and cancer.

aromatic amine class of chemical causing cancer. See *aniline dyes and *aromatic amines.

arsenic poisonous metal-like element, occurring free in nature and in minerals. Arsenical compounds were once used to treat cancer, syphilis and various skin diseases, and are still used in cases of sleeping sickness. However, salts of arsenic can cause cancer of the *skin and *lung as long as 40 years after exposure. See *chemicals as causes of cancer.

arteriosclerosis degeneration of blood vessels associated with fat deposition, which is responsible for heart disease, stroke and kidney disease. *Oral contraceptives tend to hasten the development of arteriosclerosis in young women and retard its development in post-menopausal women. The bad effect of oral contraceptives on arteriosclerosis in young women is increased by *tobacco smoking and by high blood pressure. See *breast cancer.

asbestos Men who worked in the asbestos industry were shown by the celebrated English cancer epidemiologist Sir Richard *Doll to have lung cancer 11 times more frequently than the general population. Asbestos workers who smoked were at much greater risk. Asbestos causes *lung cancer and *mesothelioma as well as the lung disease asbestosis.
   The are three major types of asbestos: blue (crocidolite), white (chrysotile) and brown (amosite). In Australia, crocidolite was mined at *Wittenoom, and there are chrysotile mines at *Baryulgil and *Barraba. White asbestos is commonly used in lagging and insulation. South African Blue Cape crocidolite asbestos is the most dangerous

13

and likely to cause a particular type of cancer, previously rare, called mesothelioma.

Asbestos is used in various building materials, including pipes, roofing, floors, chimneys, gutters, plastics and paints. Asbestos in motor vehicle clutches and brake linings still represents a compromise between utility and known health risks, However, *epidemiological studies have not shown asbestos from the latter to be a significant danger to the public, or to the mechanics who replace clutches and brake linings.

Those exposed to asbestos include miners, packers and workers in the manufacture of asbestos products. Plumbers, builders, electricians and home handymen are at risk. Asbestos locked into buildings in Australia is being removed at great cost. Unless the workers who remove the asbestos are very careful, the risk to them is great. In fact, if their safety is not guarded rigorously, there will be more cancers than would be caused if the asbestos were left locked into the buildings. It has been estimated that for the average office worker in a building that incorporated asbestos in its construction, the risk of death (predominantly from cancer) from inhalation of asbestos fibres in the office air is around one-hundredth of the risk, first, of death in a road accident while driving to work, and second, of cancer death caused by *passive smoking at work.

Since asbestos is a compound containing silica, the question arises, is there a risk from glass, which is a silica compound? Mesotheliomas can be produced by inoculating glass fibre into animals. Fortunately *fibreglass is too big to be inhaled, and studies of 25,000 glass fibre workers have shown only one death from mesothelioma. Powder produced by grinding glass is another matter and strict precautions should be taken against inhaling it. Synthetic or man-made ceramic fibres have not been associated with disease.

Besides lung cancer and mesothelioma, asbestos can cause cancer of the *larynx and it is under suspicion of causing cancers of the *pancreas.

aspartame   food additive marketed in the USA under the name *Nutrasweet, consisting of two *amino acids, aspartic acid and pheny-lalanine. It is free of cancer risks.

aspirin   drug used to relieve pain, inflammation and fever. When taken in large amounts over long periods may cause cancer of the *bladder, and *ureters.

atomic bombs and nuclear reactors   When the atomic bombs were used against Japan in 1945, no radiation effects were foreseen. It was expected that those hightly exposed would not survive the heat and the blast. The fate of 600,000 survivors of the bombing of *Hiroshima and about 30,000 survivors of the bombing in *Nagasaki showed, in the subsequent 40 years, the capacity of radiation from nuclear bombs to cause cancer.

*Leukaemia was the first cancer to show an excess among survivors of the atom bombings in Japan, and appeared a few years after the blasts. Leukaemias were also the most frequent of cancers induced by the bombs. Cancers of the *breast, *lung, *bone, *stomach and other organs occurred more frequently in those exposed to the bombs than in non-exposed subjects. Rates of *multiple myeloma rose among the survivors after a latent period of 15 years.

The increased rate of cancer in the survivors of atomic bombs has continued for at least 40 years.

Between 1952 and 1958, 21 British atmospheric nuclear bomb tests took place in the South Pacific and Australia; Britons also took part in American tests and in cleaning up operations in the same region until 1967. A survey of more than 22,000 men who took part in these tests did not prove an effect on the total risk of developing cancer, but these men do appear to be at increased risk of developing multiple myeloma and leukaemia.

There has been much debate as to whether the accident at the *Windscale nuclear reactor was responsible for an increase in cancer. There has been a high incidence of childhood leukamia in the surrounding population, but the workers in the plant, who would be more exposed to radiation than their families, are not at increased risk for the development of leukaemia.

*Epidemiological studies showed higher leukaemia mortality rates at ages 0–24 in British districts near other nuclear installations than in comparable districts not near nuclear plants, even though the environmental radiation levels around these other plants are much lower than doses expected to cause any detectable increase in leukaemia. So even in the vicinity of other nuclear plants, where the environmental radiation was lower than around *Sellafield (formerly Windscale), childhood leukaemia rates were raised.

A recent study suggested that the nuclear installations may not be to blame for this; the childhood leukaemia mortality around so-called 'phantom nuclear power stations'—that were planned but never built, or built later—was also unusually high. Unrecognized risk factors other than environmental radiation pollution could be responsible for the increased rates of childhood leukaemia at the site of the British nuclear installations.

A still more recent study raised the possibility that the increased incidence of leukaemia and also of *lymphoma among the children near Sellafield was due to irradiation of their fathers before they were conceived. Five children from Seascale, a village near Sellafield, had leukaemia. This represented a sixfold to eightfold increase above the average childhood risk of leukaemia. Three of these five had fathers who had accumulated radiation doses over 6–13 years that exceeded the recommended limits.

Atomic bombs and nuclear reactors

If the increased incidence of leukaemia in children were due to irradiation of their fathers, it has to be presumed that the irradiation affects the testicular *cells of the workers, producing *mutations in the sperm that lead to leukaemia in the children. Because of the very small number of cases in this study that supported this possibility, and as there is no other study showing such as effect in humans, more evidence is needed. No increase in leukaemia was found in 7400 children of Japanese men who survived the atomic bomb explosions, although an increase in leukaemia was found in the offspring in a study of mice in which the fathers were irradiated.

Exposure to radiation is measured in units called milliSieverts (mSv). An annual dose limit of 50 mSv for radiation workers, recommended in 1965 by the International Commission on Radiological Protection, operates in UK and Australia, although in 1987 the British National Radiation Protection Board recommended a reduction to 15mSv per year. It has been suggested, on the basis of the Sellafield findings, that the children of men most exposed to radiation at the *Olympic Dam uranium mine mine near *Roxby Downs in the far north of South Australia may be more likely to develop leukaemia than other children. Ninety per cent of workers at *Olympic Dam received 12mSv or less in 1988–9, although a few were exposed to 20–30mSv per year.

The cancer burden induced by the *Chernobyl nuclear reactor accident is yet to be determined. One estimate is that Chernobyl will add 1 cancer per 10,000 persons to the incidence of cancer in Southern Bavaria, where the incidence is already about 1 in 4 persons.

Seventeen radioactive elements were detected in Southern Bavaria in April–May 1986, after the Chernobyl accident. The most important of these are *cesium-137, *cesium-134 and *strontium-90, because of their long *half-lives of 30, 2 and 29 years respectively. *Iodine-131 was present in relatively high concentrations, but as its half-life is only 8 days, it does not represent a persistent problem. Radioactive cesium and strontium get into milk, meat and cereals. Strontium has a long biological half-life, because it is incorporated into bones instead of calcium, where it persists for a long time. Cesium is lost from the body much more quickly.

Another radiation accident occurred in *Goiânia, Brazil, in September 1987, when a discarded radiotherapy cylinder of cesium-137 was left on a rubbish tip. The cylinder was broken open and the glowing material taken from inside it was regarded as magical, carried around, rubbed on the body and eaten by many. Apart from the 4 who have died of acute radiation effects the consequences for the 244 people who were known to be contaminated will only become known over the years. This accident illustrates the consequences of laxity of controls over the use of radioactive substances.

When nuclear fuels are considered as an alternative to fossil fuels, which themselves are causing detrimental changes to the Earth's atmosphere, we must not forget the relationship of the nuclear power industry to the production of nuclear weapons.

In the USA, all commercial nuclear power plants are monitored by the Nuclear Regulatory Commission. When the Three Mile Island plant in USA came close to meltdown of its radioactive core in 1979 the details were disclosed to the public. However, facilities which produce nuclear fuels for weapons are operated by the US Department of Energy and are not subject to monitoring by the Nuclear Regulatory Commission. Some of these plants have had serious accidents. The United States and the Soviet Union have 60,000 nuclear warheads.

auramine a yellow dye used for textiles, paper and leather. Auramine O is used as a food colouring in some countries (not Australia) and as a tissue stain. There is a risk of *bladder cancer to workers engaged in the manufacture or use of auramine. See *occupation and cancer.

autologous bone marrow transplantation (ABMT) see *bone marrow transplantation.

avian lymphoma virus cause of lymphoma in chickens. See *viruses and cancer.

B

barium enema   X-ray examination of the large bowel after it has been outlined by a suspension of barium sulphate, which is opaque to X-rays. See *bowel cancer.

Barraba   *chrysotile mine in New South Wales, not associated with *mesothelioma. See *asbestos.

Baryulgil   *chrysotile mine in northern New South Wales which closed in 1979. While workers have developed lung disease, the mine has not been associated with *mesothelioma. See *asbestos.

basal cell carcinoma   type of *skin cancer

BCNU   trade name of carmustine, medication used in cancer *chemotherapy

Beasley, R. Palmer   contemporary American medical scientist and epidemiologist who proved that *hepatitis B virus is a causative factor in *liver cancer

benign tumour   accumulation of a *clone of cells, distinguished from *malignant tumour or cancer by slow growth and by not spreading via blood or lymph vessels. See *nature of cancer.

benzanthracene   cancer-inducing *polycyclic hydrocarbon

benzene   chemical in petroleum causing *leukaemia

benzepyrene   cancer-inducing *polycyclic hydrocarbon

benzidine   chemical used in the rubber industry, causing *bladder cancer

BEREAVEMENT
In Western societies about 1 person in 20 has lost a spouse and 85% of the widowed are women. The average age of these women is about 56. Only 7% remarry.

Loss of a loved person causes a series of powerful emotions. Most people suffer somewhat the same emotions, but there are big differences, depending on the age of the mourner, the cultural background, the circumstances of the loss and many other factors.

Studies of grieving persons suggest a number of stages of grief. At first there is a **phase of protest**, involving non-acceptance and denial. Some simply cannot accept that the person is dead and continue to behave as if nothing has happened. People often feel shock and loss of all emotional capacity.

Weeping is interpreted in many ways. It is a protest, a call for attention, an attempt to get the loved one to return. It is often mingled with anger and hostility towards a world that permitted the death.

After a shorter or longer time—sometimes a few months—comes the **phase of disorganization** in which awareness of the loss develops. The predominant emotion is sadness, but there is also a yearning for the return of the loved one. Depression is a natural accompaniment, but it is not normally a destructive depression in which the mourner thinks of him- or herself as worthless or evil. There is often an element of guilt which may be tinged with anger, in which there is a feeling that more should have been done for the deceased during his life.

Grieving people often feel unwell, lacking energy, suffering various aches and pains and a sense of physical exhaustion. Memories of the dead person make these sensations worse.

Often a sense of unreality develops during this time, bringing with it a strong tendency to withdraw from the world. Responses to being comforted vary from weeping to anger and hostility. Activity may be merely automatic, doing the chores but just going through the motions of living.

Preoccupation with memories and inability to accept the loss dominate this period of disorganization. Eventually the mourner has to make the transition back to life, into the **phase of reorganization**. Eventually it becomes possible to put some of the husband's clothes away, rearrange the house and make changes from the old order.

Memories fade inevitably, and the intense grief gives way to pleasurable reflections. The widow makes new initiatives, undertakes new activities, forms new friendships, but not without guilt. This so-called survivor guilt can be a very powerful impediment to making a new life. However making a new life is necessary and it entails new personal growth. This does not necessitate departure from attitudes and values that were the strength of the old relationship.

Abnormal Grief Reactions
Some bereaved persons do not have normal grief reactions. Pain and sadness may be delayed for months or years. Others may experience a prolonged period of disorganization, with profound withdrawal from society. Serious depression may ensue, accompanied by suicidal feelings, anger and loss of self esteem.

Health often declines during the period of mourning. The death rate among widows and widowers is considerably higher during the first year of bereavement than for those of the same age and sex who still have a spouse.

Beryllium

Every culture has developed ways to meet death. Many think that the rapid removal of the body that occurs in modern hospitals removes one of the important stimuli to recognition of death. Funerals help this recognition and viewing of the body in the casket may not be the barbarous ritual that some perceive it to be.

Those whose grief does not resolve normally need help. The busy doctor may find it hard, particularly if the deceased was his or her patient. Simply helping the bereaved to talk about the death may facilitate the mourning process. Foreknowledge of the emotional patterns that will ensue is a help. Reassurance that the different intense emotions are normal encourages the widow to believe that she can emerge from the pain. Reassurance about feelings of anger and guilt are particularly helpful, especially when the sufferer is being encouraged to make a new life.

*Anti-cancer societies can direct people to sources of help, including organizations dedicated to helping bereaved people.

beryllium metallic element. Beryllium and beryllium compounds are strongly suspected of being human *carcinogens. Beryllium compounds are extremely toxic. Beryllium salts are used in alloys, ceramics and electronics, and in gas mantles. Before the 1950s beryllium was used in fluorescent lights. See *occupation and cancer.

betel leaf and nut chewed in South-East Asia, causing *mouth cancer

biopsy removal of tissue from the body for examination. Material is cut out at operation or removed through tubes or hollow needless.

bischloromethyl ether member of the *chloromethyl ether class of carcinogens, an extremely powerful inducer of *lung cancer formed when hydrogen chloride and *formaldehyde are mixed

Bittner, John J. 1904–61, US biological scientist who recognized the factor in milk of mice with breast cancer, now known as *Bittner virus, which transmits the disease to suckling mice.

Bittner virus of mice named after American cancer researcher John *Bittner. The Bittner virus, transmitted through mothers' milk, causes breast cancer in mice. See *breast cancer, viruses and cancer.

BLADDER AND URETER CANCER

Tumours of the bladder and ureters often start as *polyps, *benign tumours or abnormal areas of bladder *epithelium. Often more than one tumour is found. New tumours frequently arise within a short time of removal of a benign tumour.

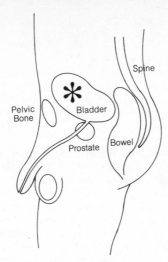

Fig. 2:

Cancer of the bladder. The urinary bladder is low in the pelvis.
It receives urine from the kidneys via the ureters (see Fig. 16).
Cancer of the bladder may spread into other structures in the
pelvis, including bones, the bowel and nerves. Cancers of the
ureters are uncommon and are similar to cancers of the bladder.

These cancers are uncommon in young people and are more often
seen after 50.

Cause of Cancer of the Bladder and Ureters
*Occupations associated with the use or manufacture of *benzi-
dine, *magenta, *naphthylamine and *auramine entail an increased
risk of bladder cancer. *Tobacco is an important factor. Between
30% and 40% of cases of cancer have been attributed to smoking and
this has been felt to be the main cause of the increase in the number
of cases of bladder cancer in the 20th century. Pain-relieving medications *aspirin and *phenacetin are also causative factors if taken in
large quantities over a long period. Heavy consumption of *coffee is
also suspected of causing these cancers. Food sweeteners have been
suspected, but the research evidence does not confirm the suspicion.

Symptoms of Bladder and Ureteric Cancers
Passing blood in the urine is usually the first sign of bladder cancer.
Sometimes there is a need to pass water frequently. Cancers of the
bladder and ureters do their damage by spreading locally. If the
cancer blocks the flow of urine from the kidney, the patient may have
*pain in the loin and may suffer effects of poor kidney function, such

21

as tiredness and *anaemia. Bladder cancer may invade nerves and bones in the pelvis, causing severe pain.

Diagnosis of Bladder and Ureteric Cancer
Bladder cancer is diagnosed by viewing the internal wall of the bladder through a *cystoscope passed through the urethra, the tube from the bladder to the exterior of the body. Examination of a *biopsy specimen confirms the diagnosis. A *pyelogram will show blockages and tumours.

Treatment of Cancer of the Bladder and Ureters
Early cancers can be removed by *surgery. Unfortunately, bladder cancers often recur or new superficial tumours arise. There are treated by putting chemotherapeutic medications into the bladder or by the Nd-YAG *laser. Widespread and recurrent bladder cancer may necessitate excision of the bladder, a decision not undertaken lightly. Some cases respond to *radiotherapy and *chemotherapy. New chemotherapeutic regimes have improved the control of bladder cancer significantly and there is recent evidence that instilling immune stimulants into the bladder may reduce recurrence. See *immunotherapy.

After treatment for bladder cancer, patients need regular urine tests for blood and cancer cells as signs of recurrence. They should also be checked regularly by *cystoscopy.

bleomycin   medication used in cancer *chemotherapy

Blenoxane   trade name of bleomycin

Bloom, David   born 1892, Warsaw-born dermatologist who migrated to the USA in 1920. Bloom worked at New York University, where he identified the disease which bears his name.

Bloom's syndrome   inherited condition in which cancers arise frequently because of a defect in the capacity of cells to repair damage to *DNA. See *heredity and cancer, *skin cancer, *mutation.

BONE CANCER
Most cancers of bone arise in other organs and spread to bone by the blood stream. A wide variety of primary tumours may spread to bones in this way. The commonest are cancers of *prostate, *breast and *lung and *lymphomas.

Osteosarcoma, Ewing's sarcoma and chondrosarcoma are uncommon primary tumours of bone. Multiple myeloma is a cancer that usually arises in the *bone marrow and causes widespread thinning or patchy destruction of bones.

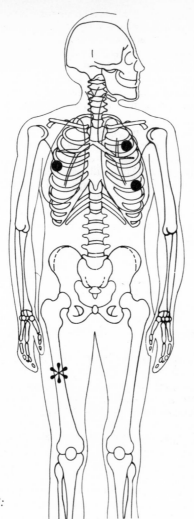

Fig. 3:

Osteosarcoma. This cancer of bone (*) arises most commonly in the femur, the bone of the upper leg. It almost invariably spreads to the lungs (●).

Bone cancer

Osteosarcoma

Osteosarcoma (or osteogenic sarcoma) occurs most commonly in older children and young adults.

Osteosarcoma in persons over 40 years of age usually occurs in *Paget's disease of bone, a disturbance of bone formation, or it results from exposure to *X-rays.

Osteosarcoma usually causes few symptoms until the primary tumour is quite advanced. The bones affected most commonly are the femur, the long bone of the upper leg, and the pelvis. Pain is the usual symptom. An aching thigh in a young person should always be investigated by X-ray, unless a satisfactory explanation is found. An X-ray usually shows typical distortion of the bone.

There are two major problems with osteosarcoma. Firstly, removal of the tumour usually involves *surgery that causes loss of the affected limb. Secondly, the tumour spreads early, so that although surgery may be effective in eradicating the primary tumour, the tumours which appear later kill the patient. These metastases are usually in the lung.

The outlook for osteosarcoma in young persons has improved markedly in recent years with the introduction of *adjuvant chemotherapy, which is drug treatment after surgery, designed to kill tiny deposits before they can develop into tumours.

Adjuvant chemotherapy is not easy for the patient to tolerate, involving not only side effects but also anxiety and uncertainty, coming after the shock of diagnosis and the blow of an operation that costs a limb.

In some cases operations have been devised that transplant bone to save the limb, or use a substitute material.

Chondrosarcoma

This cancer arises in bones of older subjects—from 40 on.

*Surgery is the proper treatment for most cases of this type of cancer. As a rule chondrosarcomas grow slowly and are slow to recur after they have been removed surgically.

Ewing's Sarcoma

Ewing's sarcoma is a bone cancer that usually occurs in the first three decades of life. It is usually located in the long bones, although this type of cancer can occur in any bone.

Ewing's sarcoma is a highly malignant tumour that is not usually cured by *surgery or *radiotherapy. However aggressive chemotherapy combined with radiotherapy has improved the survival of patients with this cancer.

Multiple Myeloma

Multiple myeloma is an uncommon cancer of white blood cells of the type which makes *antibodies. The incidence of myeloma has increased by 50% in the past 15 years, for reasons that are quite unknown. Exposure to *X-rays (see *ankylosing spondylitis) is a factor in causation of multiple myeloma and there may be a weak hereditary influence. Myeloma spreads all through the *bone marrow and weakens the bones.

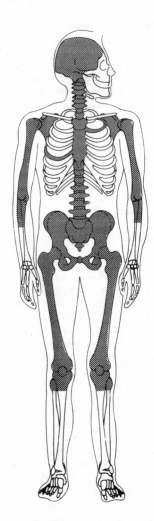

Fig. 4:

Spread of multiple myeloma. This cancer of cells of the immune system *spreads throughout the bone marrow and causes widespread thinning of bones.*

Bone marrow

*Chemotherapy offers patients with multiple myeloma a chance of good control of the disease, sometimes for several years. *Pain, a problem when bones are weakened, usually responds well to radiotherapy.

Myeloma sometimes starts as a solitary nodule, either in bone or other tissues. Such patients may be cured by *surgery combined with *radiotherapy if cancer cells have not spread to the bone marrow.

bone marrow   tissue in the cavities of bones, which gives rise to white and red blood cells. Cells can be sucked out of the marrow for examination under the microscope, or a small core of bone and marrow can be removed. Marrow is usually aspirated from the breast-bone (sternum) and cores are taken from the upper margin of the pelvic bone above the hip joint. See *bone marrow transplantation, *leukaemia, *multiple myeloma.

bone marrow transplantation   The dose of chemotherapeutic drugs that a patient can tolerate is usually limited by the poisonous effects of such drugs on cells of the bone marrow. If these cells do not recover from the side effects of *chemotherapy, the patient will die from failure to resist infections, because of a deficiency of white blood cells, from *anaemia (lack of red blood cells), or from haemorrhage, due to lack of *platelets.

To enable higher doses of chemotherapy to be given, thus giving a higher chance of cure, bone marrow may be taken out before che-motherapy, stored and transplanted into the patient after chemother-apy. This bone marrow can be obtained either from a donor or from the patient. Use of the patient's own marrow is known as *autologous bone marrow transplantation (ABMT).

Transplantation is achieved simply by putting the suspended cells into a vein, just like a blood transfusion. However, the matching of marrow has to be much more precise than the matching of blood, and incompatible marrow grafts give rise to very serious complications. Therefore there are considerable advantages to ABMT.

One unknown aspect of ABMT is the seriousness of putting back cancer cells that are in the stored marrow, after chemotherapy. There is evidence that natural defence mechanisms can kill these cells when the chemotherapy has relieved the patient of the greater proportion of his cancer. Ways of 'purging' the marrow of these cancer cells are being investigated.

It has been found recently that chemotherapy causes marrow *stem cells to leave the marrow and to circulate in the blood for a short time. Increasing use is being made of these cells, which are harvested by separating them from the blood, then returned to the patient after chemotherapy. This procedure is offering patients with cancer cells in the marrow a chance of cure.

About 15% of persons who have ABMT die from complications of the procedure, although the mortality is lower in fit persons with relatively early disease. ABMT therefore represents a lottery with extraordinarily high stakes, offering cure where other treatments do not, but with a substantial risk of death. It works best in various *leukaemias, in *Hodgkin's disease and in *lymphomas and least well in cancers which are insensitive to chemotherapy. It can only be carried out in specialized centres and its use must be considered experimental, as many aspects still need to be studied.

bone scan test for cancer deposits or other disease of bone, by detecting a *radioactive substance used as a tracer.

BOWEL CANCER

The small bowel extends from the stomach to the caecum, where the large bowel begins. The lowest part of the large bowel is the *rectum. Cancer rarely occurs in the small bowel. On the other hand, the large bowel or *colon is a common site for the development of cancer.

Worldwide, cancer of the colon and rectum is the fourth most common cancer. Colo-rectal cancers account for 13% of newly diagnosed cancers in Australia. In Western countries, 4–5% of the population have cancer of the colon, which is the second leading cause of cancer deaths in Australia and the US. This cancer accompanies a high standard of living and the highest incidence in Australia occurs in the highest *socioeconomic class—professional, executive and administrative workers. During the period 1940–65, the incidence of this cancer fell, and subsequently it has been increasing steadily. After World War II, many Italians, Greeks and Yugoslavs migrated to Australia. The longer these people have lived in Australia, the greater is the proportion of them dying from colon cancer. Large bowel cancers affect men and women approximately equally. The peak incidence is between 40 and 80 years of age.

The rectum is the site of about half of the cases of cancer of the large bowel. The incidence of rectal cancer has increased 25% in the past 10 years.

Cause of Bowel Cancer
Much of the evidence focuses on *diet as the causative factor. The relatively high incidence of the disease in beef-eating Western societies suggests that a high intake of animal *fat predisposes to the disease. This suspicion is supported by the knowledge that colon cells are the only cells of the body that can take some of their nutrition, in the form of certain fatty substances, directly from the outside world— the bowel contents. The food of all other cells comes from the bloodstream. Animal *protein has also been implicated in bowel

27

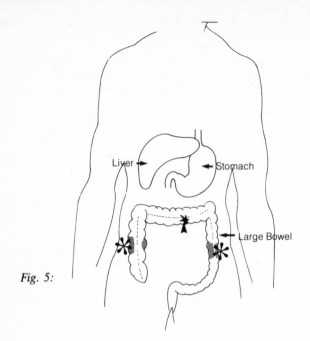

Fig. 5:

Cancer of the large bowel. Cancer may occur anywhere along the 140 cm of the large bowel (colon) and its terminal part, the rectum. Two cancers are illustrated (*) and one polyp (→). Because the contents are more fluid in the first part of the large bowel, cancer arising on the right side of the colon does not block the bowel as early as it does on the left side. A polyp *may be a precursor of a cancer.*

cancer, together with a low intake of vegetable *fibre. Deficiency of *vitamin D is also suspected to be a factor.

*Heredity plays an important part in some cases of colon cancer. The chance of having cancer of the colon is increased threefold if 1 first-degree relative has had cancer or *polyps of the colon, and nine-fold if more than 1 relative is affected.

Although the incidence of polyps has not been well documented, they occur in from 2% to 15% of the normal adult population over 50 years of age. Depending on the type of polyp, up to 30% become malignant. Unfortunately polyps commonly cause no symptoms. Sometimes they bleed, giving rise to bloody bowel motions. Uncommonly they can cause pain and disturb the bowel habit by dragging on the bowel.

*Familial adenomatous polyposis (FAP) and some other inherited intestinal polyposis syndromes are associated with an increased risk of cancer of the bowel.

Chronic inflammations of the bowel called *ulcerative colitis and *Crohn's disease also predispose to cancer of the colon. Patients who are known to be at risk of developing bowel cancer should be kept under regular surveillance by bowel examinations using *endoscopes which have been developed in the past decade.

Symptoms of Bowel Cancer

The most common symptom of bowel cancer, which often goes unheeded, is change in bowel habit. Most people have very regular bowel habits. A new habit of constipation followed by looseness of the bowels is an indication that it is time for a visit to the doctor.

Loss of blood in the motion is another cardinal warning. Blood may colour bowel motions red if the blood is lost from near the end of the bowel, but blood lost from the stomach, small bowel or upper large bowel makes the motions dark or black. Blood can easily be detected in motions by simple chemical tests. Newer tests based on antibodies are very accurate, as they are unaffected by dietary ingredients. Often bright red blood comes from *haemorrhoids (piles), but it should not be assumed that haemorrhoids are the only source of blood in the motions; if tests show blood persisting in the motions after the haemorrhoids have been treated, special examinations should be carried out to find its source.

A third finding that alerts the doctor to the possibility of bowel cancer is *anaemia. A blood test usually shows changes resulting from constant loss of blood.

Carcinoma of the colon spreads through the wall of the bowel, and travels by the *lymph stream into *lymph nodes and by the blood to the liver. Sometimes there is no recurrence after removal of lymph nodes containing metastases, but when the liver is involved, even by only a few metastases, the disease is generally incurable. Liver transplantation may help future patients with cancer deposits.

The contents of the large bowel, at first liquid, become more solid as they progress through the bowel. Blockage, causing constipation, intermittent diarrhoea and sometimes vomiting, is more frequent when the lower part of the bowel, where the contents are more solid, is affected. Cancers of the first part of the colon are often detected late because narrowing does not cause blockage of liquid faeces.

An advanced cancer may encircle the bowel, narrowing the passage, causing at first bouts of abdominal *pain and ultimately an emergency, with intractable vomiting, when the bowel is obstructed.

Diagnosis of Bowel Cancer

Bowel cancer can be found by a *barium enema. The inside of the large bowel can be observed through flexible *colonoscopes. Polyps can be removed and samples can be taken from suspicious tissue for microscopic examination. The diagnosis of bowel cancer must be confirmed by microscopic examination of tissue obtained by *biopsy.

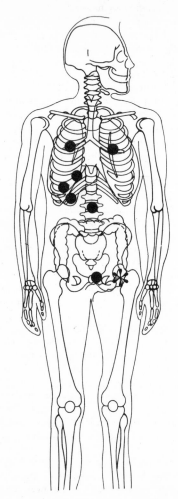

Fig. 6:

Spread of bowel cancer. Cancer of the large bowel (*) spreads directly through the bowel wall, to lymph nodes and by the blood to the liver. Early treatment offers a very good chance of removal of the cancer before it has spread.

Treatment of Bowel Cancer

If colon cancer is detected early enough, *surgery usually cures it. It is usually possible to detect large bowel cancer early, if the patient and the doctor take notice of the clues.

Colonic cancer is treated by surgery, cutting out the involved segment of the bowel. The surgeon may sometimes leave a *colostomy, that is, an opening of the bowel on the abdominal wall. A permanent colostomy is sometimes needed if the bowel cannot be rejoined after the cancer has been cut out. Sometimes the tumour is so near the end of the bowel that removal of the cancer costs the patient control of his bowel. A permanent colostomy is then necessary. Occasionally a solitary *metastasis in the liver can be removed surgically.

Some authorities favour *radiotherapy to rectal cancers before operation. *Chemotherapy may control this disease for a period of months. Infusion pumps are sometimes used to deliver a chemotherapeutic drug through a blood vessel into the liver, when that organ is involved. Sometimes very good responses are obtained, but this treatment has not led to *cures.

Table 1: Warning signs of large bowel cancer

Change of bowel habit — constipation, diarrhoea
Loss of blood in bowel motions
Anaemia — tiredness, pale skin colour

Prevention of Bowel Cancer

Currently the best advice on the avoidance of colon cancer is to reduce animal *fats and to increase *fibre in the diet. The diet should be adequate in *vitamin A. One study suggests that a high intake of the cruciferous vegetables—cauliflower, brussel sprouts, cabbage and broccoli—will reduce the risk. Another study suggests that the risk factors are a high *protein intake, a high *alcohol intake and a low *fibre intake.

*Screening for blood in the motions may improve the discovery of cancers at an early stage, greatly improving the chance of cure. Studies are being carried out in many centres to determine the value of population screening. Tests for blood in bowel motions are the only feasible and practicable way of screening populations *en masse*, but the cost may be too great for mass screening. However, selected groups of persons should be screened, namely: persons whose relatives have had bowel cancer, or a history of many cancers in the family, and persons from families which have polyps of the bowel. One opinion is that screening should begin at age 40 years, and at an earlier age if there is a family history, particularly if the cancer in the relative occurred at an early age. A new, highly specific test, which uses an *antibody to detect blood in bowel motions, can be used to monitor persons at risk of developing large bowel cancer.

Estimates vary as to the proportion of bowel cancers which do not bleed, and which would not be detected by tests for blood in the bowel motions. The proportion is probably about one third. Because of the high proportion of cancers which will not be detected this way, persons at high risk should be kept under surveillance by *colonoscopy or *X-ray.

Bowen, J.T. 1857–1941, US dermatologist, professor at Harvard from 1907, who described the type of skin cancer now named after him.

Bowen's disease type of *skin cancer. Bowen's disease may look like dermatitis or eczema, but does not respond to treatment for those conditions.

BRAIN CANCER

The brain is a common site for *secondary cancers, that arise in one organ and spread by the blood stream to the brain. The development of secondary cancers in the brain usually heralds the terminal phase of the cancer.

In the USA *primary tumours of the brain, while still not very common, have become 2 to 3 times as frequent in the past 20 years. Any kind of brain tumour, whether benign or malignant, is serious because the brain, being in a closed box, cannot expand. As the tumour grows the brain is compressed, a situation that cannot be tolerated for long.

Meningiomas are *benign tumours that arise in the membranes surrounding the brain. They can be removed successfully in most cases and do not usually regrow. They do not invade the brain. They merely compress it.

It is a tragedy if a meningioma is not diagnosed in time. The symptoms are those of brain tumours.

There are several types of *primary cancer of the brain, all causing similar manifestations. Primary cancers of the brain arise in cells which support the nerve cells, rather than in the highly differentiated nerve cells themselves. The commonest is **malignant glioma.** Unlike meningiomas, gliomas invade the brain and destroy the nerve cells.

Symptoms of Brain Tumour

The symptoms due to brain tumour are of two types. The first is headache and later vomiting, resulting from increased pressure within the skull. Symptoms of the second type result from loss of function of the part of the brain that is compressed or invaded. Some examples are loss of some of the field of vision, loss of power of limbs, and loss of awareness of one half of the body or of the world on one side of the body.

Sometimes epilepsy results, in the form of a fit in which the patient has rapid repeated involuntary movements, or an attack involving a queer sensation, or a disturbance of consciousness.

One type of benign tumour, *acoustic neuroma, causes deafness and ringing in the ears because of pressure on one of the nerves that are concerned with hearing.

Treatment of Brain Cancer

Operations inside the skull raise difficult technical problems. Even if a tumour is benign it can only be removed surgically if vital structures can be spared.

Malignant gliomas can be partially removed by *surgery if they are on the surface of the brain. However, often the removal of the tumour would cause damage to vital structures, so that operation is not possible. Malignant gliomas always recur after surgery.

In order to improve their outlook, patients with malignant glioma are usually treated with *radiotherapy after operation, and *chemotherapy is used in some centres. Despite all efforts, less than 10% of patients with gliomas survive 2 years.

BREAST CANCER

In Western countries, breast cancer is the most common malignant disease of women, accounting for 13,000 deaths annually in the United Kingdom alone. It is estimated that 7% of women in the United States will develop breast cancer during their lives. At least one Australian woman in 15 will develop the disease, which is the most common fatal cancer in young women between the age of 25 and 35 years. It is also the most common cause of death in women between the ages of 35 and 50 years. The incidence increases with age, and one third of cases occur after the age of 70 years. About 5000 new cases of breast cancer are diagnosed each year in Australia, 5 times as many as cases of *cervix cancer, and 2300 die each year of breast cancer. One per cent of breast cancers occur in men.

Cause of Breast Cancer

Several of the causative factors are known. The most potent is the female hormone *oestrogen produced by the woman's own body. Breast cancer does not occur in women who have lost their ovaries, the main source of oestrogen, in early life.

Lifestyle factors are clearly important, presumably because they affect the production of oestrogen. Early onset of periods, obesity (particularly after age 60), failure to have children, late pregnancy (at age 28 or over), late menopause and abuse of *oral contraceptives increase the risk. The onset of menstruation is probably signalled by

33

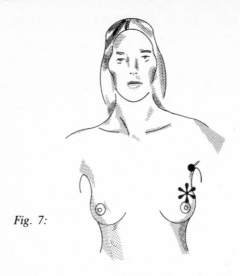

Fig. 7:

Breast cancer. Cancer of the breast usually becomes noticeable because the patient feels a lump (shown here by *). The black spot indicates a secondary deposit in a lymph gland.

the attainment of a certain body size, hence the early onset in well-nourished woman. Earlier maturation of women results in longer exposure to their own oestrogens. A greater intake of *fats provides more abundant raw materials for the production of oestrogens. Full-term pregnancy at an early age and breast feeding reduce the incidence of breast cancer in the mother.

Some authorities consider that marked social changes over recent years, resulting in women pursuing careers and postponing pregnancy, are major factors in the increase of breast cancer. It is notable that though these women are well educated, the majority still present with advanced cancers. Not simply ignorance, but denial and fear, appear to cause this to happen.

Recent studies of college women in the USA suggest quite strongly that women who were athletic in their youth are less likely to have breast cancer. At least two factors, which are probably connected, are likely to be important: a lean body and late onset of menstruation. Girls who train hard for swimming or athletics appear to start menstruating later than girls who are less active.

Breast cancer of mice is transmitted by a *virus in mothers' milk, but there is no convincing evidence of a viral cause of human breast cancer. **Heredity** evidently plays a part in some families. Ten per cent of women have a mother or sister who has had breast cancer. Women whose mothers or sisters have developed breast cancer are 2 to 3 times as likely to develop it as the female population at large. The risk is greater if a mother or sister developed primary cancers in each breast. In contrast to this minor genetic factor, major genetic differences such as exist between Japanese and Americans make no difference to the incidence of breast cancer. The relatively low incidence in Japanese women living in Japan contrasts with a high incidence in Japanese women born and living in the USA. This difference must be due to *diet or other *lifestyle factors. See *geography and cancer.

*Radiation may be a factor in causing breast cancer. The discredited practices of irradiation of the scalp of children for tinea, and irradiation of the neck and upper chest for a mythical condition of enlargement of the thymus gland, were shown in retrospect to increase the incidence of breast cancer in later life. Women who survived the *atomic bombs dropped in Japan in 1945 have an increased risk of breast cancer, especially if they were adolescent at the time they were exposed. Careful studies show that proper use of *X-rays for diagnostic purposes contributes less than 1% to the occurrence of breast cancer and this effect emerges only in the eighth decade of life.

Oral Contraceptives and Breast Cancer

Most studies have shown no increase of breast cancer in women who have used the pill. However, recent studies have suggested an increased incidence of breast cancer in childless women who take oral contraceptives over a long time before they reach the age of 25 years. Other studies suggest that taking oral contraceptives after age 45 increases the risk.

In October 1989 the US Federal Drug Administration Advisory Committee recommended that its previous ruling against the contraceptive pill for women over 35 be removed—so long as the women did not smoke. See *hormone replacement therapy.

Hormone Replacement Therapy and Breast Cancer

Use of oestrogens after the menopause reduces the thinning of bones that occurs in women as they age and reduces the development of *arteriosclerosis. These benefits have to be weighed against risk of the development of breast cancer. The best opinion today is that the benefits of oestrogen therapy outweigh the cancer risks, but the risk of breast cancer may be slightly increased. See *hormone replacement therapy.

Women should obtain a clear explanation of the benefits and risks of hormone replacement therapy from their doctors and up-to-date information on the cancer risks, before embarking on lifelong hormonal replacement.

Breast cancer

Hormone Replacement for Women who have had Breast Cancer
Women who have had a small breast cancer removed, and who had no deposits in the lymph glands that were removed at operation, have a 70% chance of cure. Hormone replacement is generally not advised for these patients, although the position is obscure. The concern is that oestrogen will encourage the growth of silent tumour cells. A blanket embargo on hormone substitution can be said to disadvantage three-quarters of these women for the potential benefit of the other quarter. Hormones may be justified in individual cases.

Symptoms of Breast Cancer
Breast cancer is first noticed by most patients as a painless lump. Another sign is a change in appearance of the nipple, sometimes resembling dermatitis. The latter condition, called *Paget's disease of the breast, usually results from cancer cells spreading from a tumour deeper in the breast.

Breast pain is not a symptom of breast cancer. Discharge from the nipple requires a visit to the doctor, but is uncommonly a sign of breast cancer. Both of these are causes of false alarms causing much anxiety.

Advanced breast cancer associated with tumours in bones may cause *pain. Curiously, although *bone scans and X-rays may alert the doctor to deposits of breast cancer in bone, patients often experience no pain. If nerves are pressed on, or bones fracture, pain is usually felt, but it is not known why bones involved with cancer are sometimes painful and sometimes not. If the liver is involved the patient loses energy. If the brain is involved, the symptoms are those of *brain cancer.

Diagnosis of Breast Cancer
Diagnosis of breast cancer is usually made by obtaining a core of tumour tissue by needle *biopsy. After other tests, including a *bone scan, have been completed, the situation is discussed fully with the patient, who may agree to operation if it is advised. These tests usually include a scan of bone for spots of cancer, using a radioactive tracer substance.

Early Detection of Breast Cancer
Although other methods have been developed to detect breast cancer at an early stage, there are only three ways that are really practicable: examination of breasts by women themselves, examination by a doctor, and *mammography.

When a woman feels what she believes to be a lump, she should not immediately conclude that it is a cancer. Many lumps are *benign. Many can quickly be shown to be cysts, by examination of the cyst fluid taken out through a fine hollow needle by the surgeon.

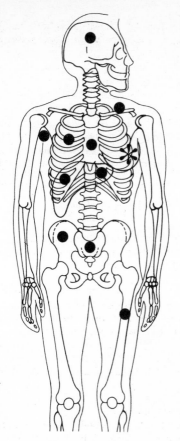

Fig. 8:

  *Spread of breast cancer. Seedlings from the primary tumour
(*) may become tumours in lungs, bones, liver, brain and skin.*

Breasts in menstruating women develop lumpiness as the month
proceeds.

Breast Self-examination
There are a number of techniques that women may use to find a
breast lump early. The important points are that the examination
should be carried out regularly, using one of the reliable techniques,
and for menstruating women should take place a few days after the
menstrual period each month.

Breast cancer

Some people feel that such a preoccupation with breast lumps would bring about a state of great anxiety in many women and that the stress would be unbearable if a lump were found. Since most lumps are not cancers, they argue, many unnecessary visits to the doctor would result. There are also conflicting reports on the efficacy of breast self-examination.

In one technique of breast self-examination called the 'strip method', the breast and the surrounding tissues are divided into an imaginary map. Each 5 cm spot on the map grid is felt using a rotary motion of the flat of the hand, first with light then with deep pressure.

Women with small breasts can examine them standing in the shower or lying down. Women with large breasts should examine them when lying down.

Table 2: Ways to detect breast cancer early

Breast self-examination

Expert examination by a doctor

Mammography

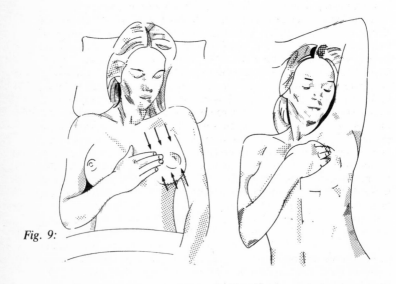

Fig. 9:

Breast self-examination. All women should develop the habit of examining their breasts regularly for lumps. The illustration shows the technique for examination on the bed (left) and self-examination in the shower (right).

The right breast is examined with the left hand, after placing the right hand behind the head. The positions are reversed for examining the left breast. The outer halves of the breast are examined more easily with a pillow under the head. The armpit should be included in the examination. For examination of the nipple area and the inner half of the breast, it is best to remove the pillow to flatten the inner half of the breast.

The examination must include an inspection in the mirror, to look for dimpling, puckering of the skin, or irregularities. Pulling in of or discharge from the nipple should not be missed. Breasts are never symmetrical, but they retain their shapes and relative positions. In other words, if, for example, the breast which usually reaches lower changes its position relative to the other breast, this should be further investigated.

Most *Anti-Cancer Societies issue illustrated instructions for breast self-examination. The available evidence suggests that lives are saved through finding tumours by breast self-examination, but examination of the breast by either the woman or her doctor is less effective at finding lumps than mammography.

Mammography
Mammography is a special type of *X-ray examination.

A big and expensive trial, the UK Trial of Early Detection of Breast Cancer, illustrates difficulties in obtaining irrefutable proof of the value of screening for breast cancer. In this trial, women aged 45–64 were enrolled between 1979 and 1981, and observed for 7 years: 54,841 women were screened by physical examination annually and had mamography in alternate years; 63,636 were offered teaching in breast self-examination and were provided with a self-referral clinic. The results in these two groups of women were compared with the outcome in 127,117 women for whom no extra services were provided. The risk of dying from breast cancer was 14% less in the two groups of women offered screening. The groups were not exactly comparable, but even when calculations included allowances for differences between the two groups, such as age, the reduction was not more than 20%. Although the numbers of subjects are very large, these differences fall short of true statistical significance.

Despite the failure of this trial to achieve results of statistical significance, its findings have been used to support screening of breast cancer. Other trials in the USA and Sweden have shown a reduction of 30% in the death rate over a period of 5 years in women who have been screened by mammography for breast cancer. However, careful analysis indicates that the reason these women survived was less fatal disease of other kinds, rather than early detection and treatment of breast cancer. No benefit can be shown with mammography in women under 50 years of age (possibly because tumours are more difficult to detect in younger women).

Breast cancer

In advising women to have mammography, it should not be forgotten that there is a radiation risk from mammography which may actually cause some breast cancers. However, the technology has advanced so that mammography now uses much lower doses of X-rays than most diagnostic X-ray procedures. On the positive side, cancers found by mammographic surveys are on average smaller than those coming to notice in other ways. It is now claimed that more than 90% of breast cancers can be detected by mammography, most of them before a lump can be felt, and that the earlier detection afforded by the latest mammographic techniques substantially improves the outcome, beyond the 70% 5-year cure rate quoted for surgery of early cases. Occasionally a breast cancer is detected by palpation before it can be seen by mammography.

Women under 40 years should not have routine mammograms, because abnormalities are hard to detect, the breasts of young women being more dense to X-rays. Mammographic abnormalities are easier to detect in women more than 50 years of age.

Like other tests, mammography is not 100% accurate. Sometimes lumps that prove later to be cancers do not show up on mammography. The danger of a lump not showing on mammography is greater in young women. If any lump persists in a premenstrual woman over more than one menstrual cycle, she needs a specialist examination even if the mammogram is negative.

The best advice that can be given at present is that women over the age of 50 should probably have mammography every one or two years. Governments are currently grappling with the problems of setting up mass screening facilities.

In Australia, public and private, static and mobile breast screening units from all States are involved in Commonwealth evaluation of screening programmes. The estimated cost per examination in this programme is $A15 and it has been claimed that early detection targeted at women over 40 could lead to a 16% reduction in deaths, a saving of 370 lives a year.

About 10% of women in Australia with a breast lump neglect it and eventually seek medical help with advanced cancer. This proportion remains constant for women of all *socioeconomic classes and levels of education. The reason for not seeking medical advice is, in most cases, fear of losing the breast rather than lack of knowledge.

Treatment of Breast Cancer

The aim of treatment is to cure if possible, Small primary breast cancers are treated by *surgery.

If, unfortunately, clinical examination and special tests confirm that the cancer has spread to lungs, liver, bone marrow, other vital organs, or to skin, cure is not possible at present. Treatment by *radiotherapy, *chemotherapy or both is then needed.

Removal of a breast can only be justified by the intention to cure. An exception to this rule is the case of big tumours that would cause great trouble if allowed to persist. These cases are usually treated by radiotherapy and/or chemotherapy first, to reduce the size of the operation.

Today many patients are offered an operation, a so-called *lumpectomy, which removes the segment of the breast which is involved by the tumour. Later, the operation site is treated by radiotherapy. Alternatively, a plastic operation (*mammaplasty) may enable a breast to be reconstructed. These patients are spared the great psychological damage caused by mastectomy.

Surgery cures about 50% of all patients, but 70% of early cases are cured. Surgery often fails because cancer cells have travelled to other parts of the body and have established new cancer colonies. Even when breast cancers are small, they sometimes spread by the *lymph and the blood streams. In such cases tumours appear at any time after the operation, even more than 20 years later.

It is actually incorrect to speak of recurrence in most of these cases. Tumours appearing after the operation result from distant spread of tumour cells before the operation. Such seedlings may be only a few cells, and are therefore quite undetectable by any means. Why they lie dormant, and conversely, why they start growing after many years, is not known. The same phenomenon is seen in other tumours, such as *malignant melanoma and *kidney cancer.

It may not be necessary or helpful to remove the breast if preoperative tests show that the disease has spread so far that no cure is possible. Then the patient may be offered treatment including chemotherapy, followed by radiotherapy or limited operation.

Patients who must have mastectomy will find a mastectomy service in the *Anti-cancer Society in their capital city. This service, staffed by women who have gone through the loss of a breast, can help women overcome the stresses of mastectomy.

Recurrence of breast cancer is treated with *hormones, by *chemotherapy, and by *radiotherapy.

Hormonal Treatment of Breast Cancer

The side effects of hormone treatment are usually minimal, but not all cases respond to hormone treatment, and the duration of response is variable. It is standard practice to test the tumour for hormone *receptors at the time of operation, in case the cancer recurs. Cancers that are positive in receptor tests usually respond to treatment with each kind of hormone—*oestrogen, *androgen, *progestin—and *tamoxifen which is a hormone inhibitor. Furthermore, when relapse occurs during the first hormone treatment, there is a good chance of a second or third response by changing the hormone. A successful second-line strategy is to block the production of hormones, including

Breast cancer

oestrogen, by the adrenal gland, with a drug called *aminoglutethimide. As production of the essential *cortisone type hormones is also
blocked, patients on aminoglutethimide must always take an effective
form of cortisone by mouth, at all times. If they become sick, have an
accident or an operation, they will need more, not less, cortisone.

Chemotherapy in Breast Cancer
Most women dread the thought of *chemotherapy, but are very
grateful for its beneficial effects. Low-toxicity chemotherapy gives
good control to many women, and the side-effects are usually quite
acceptable in the light of the benefits. After overcoming their initial
dread, these women experience improved wellbeing and control of
symptoms. Regimes with higher doses and more toxic drugs give a
better chance of long-term control, with greater risk of complications.
These decisions must be made by the patient with her doctor after
consultation and explanation.

Radiotherapy in Breast Cancer
*Radiotherapy may be used in association with excision of the
primary tumour and in the control of symptoms. Bone pain responds
well to radiotherapy.

Adjuvant Chemotherapy for Breast Cancer
Even in the most favourable circumstances, the risk of recurrence
of breast cancer is 30%. There is also a 1% risk per year of the
development of a new breast cancer in women who have had treatment for breast cancer.

'Adjuvant chemotherapy' is used here to include antihormonal
treatment as well as cytotoxic drugs. Cyclical *chemotherapy with
cytotoxic drugs is used to reduce rates of relapse in premenopausal
patients with breast cancer, and *tamoxifen is used in postmenopausal women. The chemotherapy is commonly carried on for 6 months
Opinions differ on the optimal duration of treatment with tamoxifen.

Large *clinical trials have shown that the risk of recurrence of
breast cancer can be reduced by about 20% or more when chemotherapy is used as an adjuvant to surgery, depending on factors
like age and spread to lymph nodes. This is equivalent to an increase
of 6–10% in the number of subjects surviving 5 years after the inital
treatment. Unfortunately, nobody knows which breast cancers have
disseminated by the time of diagnosis and treatment. In those in
whom the malignant cells have spread to other parts of the body, the
cells may remain dormant for 20 or 30 years and many women will
live out their lives before tumours become apparent. The main indica-
tor of distant spread in those who have no apparent metastases is
seedlings in the lymph nodes in the axilla—the armpit. If positive
nodes are discovered the patient is likely to be offered adjuvant or

prophylactic treatment. Women who have not yet passed the menopause are usually given chemotherapy, and post-menopausal women receive tamoxifen.

As well as preventing the emergence of metastases, tamoxifen may prevent the development of new breast cancers. In this respect the drug may be the forerunner of medications for *chemoprevention, that is, use of medications to prevent the development of cancer.

The decision to use adjuvant chemotherapy with cytotoxic drugs is not reached lightly, because of its side effects. A proportion of women will receive treatment which they do not need. There is no way around this dilemma while it remains impossible to pick those who may benefit from the adjuvant chemotherapy.

Prevention of Breast Cancer

We have seen that dietary factors are strongly suspected of causing the high incidence of breast cancer in Western women. Unfortunately, the dietary factors at work have not been clearly identified. In these circumstances, the only advice that can be given is to eat a sensible diet, exercising restraint in the amount of animal *fat consumed. Animal meats and fats make an obvious difference between Western and Japanese diets and this may help to explain the lower incidence of breast cancer among women eating traditional Japanese food. The case against *alcohol as a minor factor seems conclusive, and the intake of alcohol before the age of 30 years is most important. Girls should be encouraged to take an active part in sport, and to watch their diets, as part of a programme to avoid early onset of menstruation.

bronchoscope   rigid or flexible *endoscope for examining the airways of the lung.

bronchoscopy   endoscopic examination of the airways

Burkitt, Denis   born 1907, Irish-British surgeon who worked in the colonial service in Africa and described the *lymphoma which bears his name. Burkitt also drew attention to the relationship of bulky stools resulting from a high *fibre diet to the low incidence of *bowel cancer in Africans.

Burkitt's lymphoma   Burkitt's lymphoma is of particular theoretical importance because the *Epstein-Barr virus is a causative factor in the development of this tumour in Africa, yet the same virus affects virtually everybody in other parts of the world without causing cancer. Burkitt's lymphoma is frequent only in restricted geographical zones in Africa, which overlap the malaria belt, and the incidence is greatest near lakes, below an altitude of 1500 m, suggesting that malaria is an essential cofactor in causing the lymphoma.

Butter yellow

Besides affecting *lymph nodes, these tumours affect the jaws of young children and the ovaries of girls. *Chemotherapy cures a proportion of cases.

butter yellow   *aniline dye. See *chemicals as causes of cancer.

C

cadmium metallic element considered capable of causing cancer. Recent *epidemiological studies indicate that cadmium as used in industry today is not responsible for *prostate cancer. Although workers exposed to cadmium appear to have increased mortality from *lung cancer, other factors may contribute to this. See *metals.

caesium see *cesium

caffeine Caffeine is found in *coffee, *tea, *cocoa and cola drinks. It is stimulant of the brain, muscles, heart and circulation.

A number of surveys have raised the possibility of an association between caffeine and cancer. Prominence given by the press to these surveys has caused unnecessary alarm.

There is no good evidence to link caffeine to any human cancer, including cancer of the *bladder and cancer of the *pancreas.

cancer-inducing chemicals in food Most prepared foods that we buy, and many raw foods, contain additives. More than 1500 chemical substances are authorized for addition to foods an Australia has an approved system of labelling for additives in packaged foods. The additives are designated by numbers on the package. The code numbers can be translated with the aid of a readily available 'code breaker'. See the reference list contained in the Appendix.

Our food undoubtedly contains pesticide residues, including the *chlorinated insecticides which have been banned in most countries. It is impossible to assess their potential to induce cancer, or to provide a balanced view on avoidance of food produced with the use of chemical fertilizers and pesticides.

New compounds are introduced from time to time to expedite growth—*hormones in meat production and plant *growth factors for the production of fruit and vegetables.

*Daminozide is one such recent product which is used in apple orchards to regulate growth of the trees and to intensify the colour of red apples before harvest. It has been reported to have cancer-producing potential in mice, but whether it is dangerous to humans is yet to be proved. See *chemicals as causes of cancer.

cancer screening see *screening for cancer, *breast, *cervix, *bowel, *lung, *prostate cancers

cancer warning signs see *warning signs of cancer

carbohydrate class of food, made up of sugar-type units, distinct from *protein and *fat. Sugars, starch and vegetable *fibres are

45

carbohydrates. Carbohydrates are digested in the bowel into their sugar components and absorbed in that form. In the body they are used for energy or stored in the liver and muscles as sugar complexes.

carcinogen   agent that causes cancer. A carcinogen is defined scientifically as any substance, organism or physical agent that acts as a dominant factor in increasing the incidence of a particular kind of cancer. The three major classes of carcinogens are *chemicals, *radiations and *viruses.

carcinogenesis   process of induction of cancer, by *chemicals, *viruses and *radiations. See *causes of cancer.

carcinoma   general name for cancers arising in *epithelia, i.e. cells lining body surfaces. See *names of cancers.

carmustine   medication used in cancer *chemotherapy

carotene   family of substances in plants from which the body makes *vitamin A.

CAUSES OF CANCER
In most cases there is no single cause of cancer. A number of factors are at work. When we speak of causation of cancer, we are usually rather inaccurate, because in most cases we refer to the dominant factor. An agent that causes cancer is acting like a seed in soil. If the soil is right, the seed with take hold readily. *Carcinogens are agents that increase the incidence of cancer.

Having epidemiological evidence on age, *geographical distribution of cancer and factors in *lifestyle that influence the causation of cancer, backed up by laboratory studies, we can now define the types of agents that cause cancer. The main classes of carcinogen are *chemicals, *radiations and *viruses. More than one agent or factor is involved in causing most cancers.

Similarly we recognize *age, *heredity and *gender as factors that increase or reduce the risk of cancers developing. These factors define the soil on which cancer-inducing agents work.

As with other illnesses, cancer has to be seen as a macabre lottery. We can predict how many people will contract cancer in a population, but we cannot specify who they will be. However, we can assess the risks for a given person. Some greatly increase their number of tickets in the cancer lottery by their *lifestyle.

No cancer-inducing agent or predisposing factor claims 100% of those exposed as victims. By virtue of their heredity, constitution or other factors, some people are more resistant and some are more susceptible than the average. In terms of the lottery, tickets are allotted according to *heredity, *lifestyle and *diet.

Many people refer to a venerable ancestor who smoked rank *tobacco all his life and was killed by lightning at the age of 90. Smoking, they say triumphantly, very definitely did not kill him and from this they deduce that smoking is harmless. At the other extreme, a victim of *lung cancer, who led a blameless life and never touched a cigarette, is quoted as proof that tobacco could not possibly blamed for cancer.

By smoking, one is taking tickets in the lung cancer lottery. The more one smokes, the more chances (tickets in the lottery) one has of developing lung cancer. The non-smoker may have 1 ticket in a lung cancer lottery of 100,000 tickets. The very heavy smoker holds a third or more of all the tickets in his personal lung cancer lottery. Other factors give smokers more tickets, for example working with *asbestos. With tobacco come tickets in other cancer lotteries at the same time.

*Gender, whether you are male or female, is obviously a factor in the development of many types of cancer, for example cancer of the *breast. Breast cancer does occur in males, but it is rare. The difference between the incidence in females and males is determined by female hormones.

The lottery changes each year as we get older. For example, there are a number of childhood cancers which occur very rarely in adults. In general, however, the incidence of the common cancers increases with age.

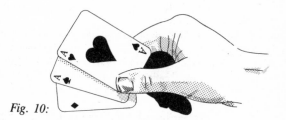

Fig. 10:

Causation of cancer. Cancer results from playing a game of chance. Everybody is in the game, because everybody is exposed to some of the risk factors. Some are at greater risk than others – in effect spending much more time at the gaming table than others. The greater the exposure to cancer-inducing agents, the greater the chance of developing cancer. Some escape, despite indulging in high-risk habits, and some whose risk appears small develop cancer. No single risk factor causes cancer in 100% of those exposed and those who have no apparent exposure to a high risk factor sometimes develop cancer.

Causes of cancer

In the past, evidence that a substance caused cancer came from observation of the groups of people in whom particular cancers occurred. Proof is obtained today in rigorous *epidemiological studies, supported by animal tests and laboratory investigations. In the past, many have died before a chemical has been proved to cause cancer. The time from exposure to developed cancer can be up to 40 years, ensuring a large number of victims of a cancer-inducing substance before effective action can stop others being exposed. The long lead time between exposure to the causative agent and the development of a recognizable tumour, in other words a long dormant period, makes identification of the causes of cancer difficult.

Cancer took five or more years to develop in Japanese victims of the *atomic bombs and cancers are still appearing in the victims more than 40 years later. During most of the interval between irradiation and the appearance of *leukaemia or cancers, there are no signs of tumour. This interval is thought to be evidence that more than one factor is often necessary for the development of a cancer. The X-rays are considered to be an *initiator, while other factors are *promoters of cancer. *Tobacco contains chemicals which are initiators and others which are promoters. This may explain why tobacco increases the risk of so many types of cancer. One or other initiator sows the seed in a cell and tobacco as the promoter waters the crop over the years.

Today, new chemical compounds are tested in experimental animals for their carcinogenic potential, and by the *Ames test, which detects changes in the growth and function of microorganisms, resulting from *mutations induced by carcinogenic compounds in their genetic material, *DNA.

The use of new chemicals is continually creating new risks. *Asbestos, *benzene and *vinyl chloride monomer are examples of industrial chemicals which killed workers until the hazards were recognized.

*Ultraviolet light causes skin cancer. The other kinds of radiation that cause cancer are the unavoidable *cosmic rays, and the relatively new hazards of *X-rays and the rays emitted by *radioactive chemicals, *atomic bombs and nuclear reactors and *radon under houses. It has been estimated that 1–2% of all fatal cancers may be caused by unavoidable, background radiations.

As with other forms of material progress, the use of radiation confers great advantages while it poses potential disadvantages of disastrous proportions. There is no safe dose of X-rays. The smallest dose confers a tiny risk and the risks from each irradiation are cumulative. The benefits associated with medical uses of X-rays and radioactive substances far outweigh the risks and these risks are being reduced by the use of better equipment and strict regulation of their use. See *medical treatment as a cause of cancer.

*Viruses are causative factors in a number of human cancers. The biggest killer is the *hepatitis B virus, causing *liver cancer, in underdeveloped countries where the incidence of hepatitis is high. The *Epstein-Barr virus is involved in causing *Burkitt's lymphoma (but only in certain geographical regions) and *nasopharyngeal carcinoma. *Adult T cell leukaemia is caused by the *human T cell leukaemia virus-I. *Human papilloma viruses are involved in the causation of *cervix cancer, a very significant çause of death from cancer in women.

Getting old is not the major factor in the development of cancer, nor is cancer inherited in most cases. Most authorities now believe that 75% or more of cancer is determined by *lifestyle and the *environment. When lifestyle and environmental factors are analyzed, the major components are *chemicals, *radiations, *viruses and *diet. There is little doubt that cancer is determined largely by where one lives, what one eats, sexual and reproductive practices, the hazards of one's work and 'recreational' drugs—particularly *tobacco and to a much lesser extent *alcohol. By controlling these factors, the burden of cancer could be reduced to one quarter of the current incidence. See *ageing and cancer, *heredity and cancer.

The incidence of cancer depends more on where and how people live than their constitutional makeup. Of countries where accurate records are kept, Scotland has the highest death rate from cancer (275 per 100,000), compared to a 217 in USA, 190 in Japan and 172 in New Zealand. The striking difference in cancer incidence between Scots and New Zealanders highlights the importance of environment or lifestyle, rather than hereditary constitution, since many people in these two populations share a common ancestry. See *geographical distribution of cancer.

The epidemiological evidence strongly suggests that *diet is a large factor in causation of *breast cancer. Whether a virus will be shown to play a part in causing this very serious disease of Western women remains to be seen. Nutrition could be acting in several ways to cause the high rate of cancer of the breast in Western societies.

Diet seems also to be the likely explanation of the increased risk of development of cancer of the *ovary, *uterus (endometrium), and *prostate in migrants from low-risk to high-risk countries.

In 1975, *stomach cancer was the most common malignant tumour in the world, but its incidence is declining everywhere, possibly as a result of better methods of storing food and of a greater consumption of fresh vegetables. These factors may work in two ways: better storage of food and refrigeration reduce the content of cancer-causing chemicals like *nitrosamines in the food, and fresh vegetables supply *carotenes and *vitamins that protect against *carcinogens.

*Bowel cancer is not declining in the Western world. Diet is thought to be the most important factor, and *fat, particularly in red meat and lack of vegetable *fibre are suspected. It will be very informative to follow the incidence of cancer in the Japanese as they increase their consumption of red meat.

Causes of cancer

Much of what we know about the incidence and causation of individual cancers in Western societies is summarized in Table 3.

Table 3: Risk factors for different cancers

Cancer	Risk Factors
Lung	Tobacco, asbestos, polycyclic hydrocarbons, arsenic, nickel, chromium, cadmium, radon, X-rays, foundry gases
Large bowel	Diet (meat, fat, lack of fibre?)
Breast	Oestrogen, early onset of periods, late menopause, late first birth, obesity, diet (fat?)
Prostate	Diet (meat, fat?), cadmium?
Stomach	Diet, low socioeconomic class, poor food preservation
Pancreas	Tobacco
Bladder	Tobacco, aniline dye products and other chemicals
Ovary	Few or no children, early onset of periods, late menopause, obesity, diet (?), decreased by oral contraceptives
Lymphoma	Impaired immune defences, Epstein-Barr virus, HTLV-I
Oesophagus	Tobacco, alcohol, nutritional deficiency (vitamin A)
Leukaemia	X-rays, benzene, chlorinated insecticides(?), Down's, Bloom's and other rare syndromes, HTLV-I virus
Kidney	Tobacco, aniline dye products, analgesics (phenacetin, aspirin)
Cervix	Papilloma virus, multiple sexual contacts, sexual partners having same, hygiene (?), tobacco
Uterus (Endometrium)	Few or no children, early onset of periods, late menopause, oestrogens unopposed by progesterone, obesity, decreased by oral contraceptives
Melanoma	Ultraviolet light, decreased skin pigment, polychlorinated biphenyls (?)
Skin	Ultraviolet light, decreased skin pigment, arsenic, X-rays, tar, mineral oils, other chemicals
Liver	Alcohol, hepatitis B virus, aflatoxin

Fig. 11:

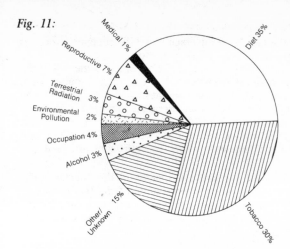

Medical 1%
Reproductive 7%
Terrestrial Radiation 3%
Environmental Pollution 2%
Occupation 4%
Alcohol 3%
Other/ Unknown 15%
Tobacco 30%
Diet 35%

*Relative importance of factors causing cancer. These figures
are based on the best epidemiological estimates. The estimates of
risks of tobacco, alcohol and terrestrial radiation (cosmic rays,
radon, ultraviolet light) are considered reliable. Risks of
occupation, air and water pollutions and medical treatment are
best estimates based on data. The others, including, diet, are
deduced or guessed estimates. "Reproductive" refers to the effect
of hormones, reproductive and sexual behaviour on development
of cancers of the breast, ovary and uterus (endometrium) and
possibly of prostate. The figures are derived from Doll, in
"Preventing Cancer", editor Tattersall, see Appendix.*

cells The existence of cells could only be recognized when micro-
scopes became available and it was not until the 1820s that the idea
was proposed that plants and animals were made of cells (see
*Schleiden, *Schwann). For a few more decades people could not
grasp where cells came from, until the great German pathologist
*Virchow pronounced that 'all cells come from other cells'. Without
this dictum there could be no progress towards modern ideas about
growth and cancer.

The cell is the basic unit of all living organisms—from animals and
plants down to single-cell animals, bacteria and viruses. The cell is the
smallest form of life that can exist independently. It is the functioning
unit of every *tissue.

Ten thousand billion cells make up an adult human. This number is
all the more remarkable when it is considered that each person starts
as one cell.

Cells

A cell can be compared to a workshop or factory.

*Enzymes are the factory's tools, facilitating the chemical processes of the cell, using energy from sugars and fats.

Information from nearby and distant cells comes to the cell in the form of specific chemical compounds or electrical impulses from nerves. Even in the case of nerves, the message from the nerve end comes in the form of a chemical released by the nerve. These chemicals deliver their messages by binding to structures on cell membranes, called *receptors. When the receptor is occupied, a chain reaction sends a signal to the *nucleus, where the messages are read and processed.

The administration of the cell takes place in the *nucleus. The nucleus is constantly responding to information from the world outside the cell. If it receives no messages the factory remains inactive. All of the documentation and workshop manuals in the nucleus are written in *DNA code.

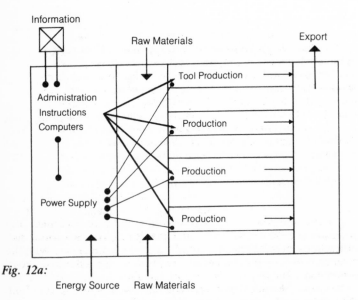

Fig. 12a:

The cell as a factory. Like a factory, a cell takes in raw materials, requires energy, receives information and needs an administration to coordinate its activities. The administration takes place in the nucleus, where the information is stored, in the form of DNA.

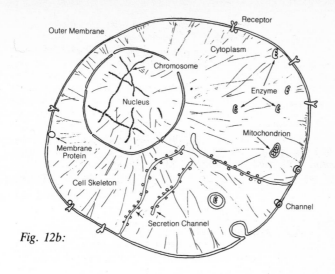

Fig. 12b:

A typical cell. This is a cross-section of a basic cell. There is an outer membrane, a nucleus and cytoplasm between the nucleus and the outer membrane. Large numbers of enzymes, tools for performing chemical reactions, drawn here much out of scale, are found in the cytoplasm. Mitochondria supply chemical energy units. The fibres making the skeleton of the cell are shown as fine lines. A pocket forming in the outer membrane will engulf particulate material and then pinch off to move into the cytoplasm. A sac which has formed in this way is present in the adjacent cytoplasm. It contains enzymes for the digestion of engulfed particles.

A computer is a remarkably good analogy of the nucleus. The computer is endowed with a programme. It receives information and instructions from the world outside it through the keyboard. The computer uses its programmes to respond to new information and instructions. The response is electrical impulses in some form of code, or language. The nucleus of a cell receives chemical information from the outside world, processes it using the DNA programmes it inherited, and responds in a chemical language, called RNA.

The *cytoplasm is the cell's workshop or factory floor. It contains the machinery for the chemical processes of the daily work of the cell. The machinery for decoding the blueprint and for copying the blueprint when the cell divides is in the nucleus.

The cell's products for export may be foodstuffs, raw materials, or processed chemicals—*growth factors, *hormones or other compounds, or excitatory substances produced by nerve cells. The chemicals released by nerves at the end of long nerve fibres activate muscles or other nerve cells.

CERVIX CANCER

Cancer of the cervix is the second most common cancer in women worldwide and the most common female cancer in developing countries. In developed countries it is the tenth most common cancer, considering both men and women. About 14,000 American women develop cervical cancer each year. The operative factor is probably venereal infection by the *papilloma virus.

Cause of Cancer of the Cervix

Cancer of the cervix does not occur in virgins. More than 200 years ago *Ramazzani of Padua observed that cervical cancer is less common in nuns than in married women. The more children a woman has, the greater the chance she has of developing cervical cancer.

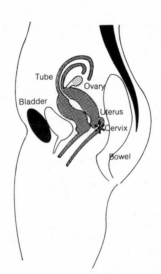

Fig. 13:

Cancer of the cervix. The cervix is the lowest part of the uterus (the womb) where it joins the vagina. The uterus empties through the cervix, and the sperm reach the ova by travelling up the cervical canal. Cancer of the cervix (*) tends to spread to neighbouring structures such as the bladder and the bowel.

Epidemiologists have determined that this cancer is more frequent the younger the age of first sexual intercourse. It is also more frequent in women of low *socioeconomic class.

Poverty is often associated with early onset of sexual activity. In a study in New York two decades ago, the incidence in Jewish women was found to be 4.7 per 100,000. In other white women it was 17.1. The incidence was very much greater in Negro (53.6) and Puerto Rican women (109.8). The incidence in Indian women is also high, whereas the lowest incidence in the world is in Israel. Circumcision and the strict rules governing sexual life of Jews probably determine the low incidence in Jewish women. The chance of developing cervical cancer is also increased by sexual promiscuity. The more sexual partners a woman has, the higher the incidence of cervical cancer. It appears that sexually promiscuous male partners can acquire and transmit the papilloma virus infection.

Cancer of the Cervix and Papilloma Virus
At least 5 types of *papilloma virus appear to be leading culprits in cancer of the cervix. Studies of women with precancerous conditions show that about 90% of abnormal cervical cells and 80% of cancer cells harbour the virus in masked form. However only a small proportion of women infected with papilloma virus go on to develop cancer.

Papilloma virus ranks as the most common sexually transmitted infection. American studies show that as many as 80% of sexually active teenage girls are infected with a cancer-causing type of papilloma virus.

The papilloma virus has also been found in cancers of the *penis. Thus cancers of the cervix and penis can be regarded as venereal diseases. It is not clear why so few males have cancer of the penis, if they harbour the virus. *Tobacco smoking and *passive smoking are both factors which increase the incidence of carcinoma of the cervix.

Oral Contraceptives and Cervical Cancer
It has proved very difficult to carry out properly controlled studies to assess the effect of *oral contraceptive pills on the incidence of carcinoma of the cervix. A number of studies do suggest that the pill slightly increases the risk of carcinoma of the cervix.

Most studies have not taken into account other risk factors, such as papilloma virus infection, smoking, multiple sexual partners and early age of first intercourse.

Diet and Cancer of the Cervix
While papilloma virus, tobacco and possibly oral contraceptives are major factors in causing carcinoma of the cervix, many researchers consider that deficiency of *vitamins A and *C are important cofactors. One study of cervix cancer has shown low levels of vitamin C in women who smoke.

Cervix cancer

Symptoms of Cancer of the Cervix

Cancer of the cervix begins, usually in women in their 20s and 30s, as a small, thin layer of abnormal cells, that can be removed completely. At this stage it causes no symptoms. However, this is the stage at which both detection and treatment are simple and effective.

Technically, early abnormalities are classified into grades of *CIN (cervical intraepithelial neoplasia), a term which has replaced the older terms *dysplasia and *carcinoma in situ. All patients with CIN should be treated.

At later stages the cancer cells wander deeper into the uterus, and later still they migrate to surrounding tissues and lymph nodes. If not treated, cancer of the cervix may come to notice because of a discharge or bleeding. These signs of the cancer occur relatively late in the disease, when it may often be incurable.

Treatment of Cervix Cancer

Cervical intraepithelial neoplasia (CIN) is treated by *surgery, *laser therapy, *diathermy, or *cryotherapy (freezing). All of these methods are very effective, producing cures in 95% of patients at the first application. The function of the ovaries and sexual function are preserved and such treatment does not impair fertility.

More advanced disease may require *surgery. *Radiotherapy can cure a proportion of later cases and can be used in older women if there are contra-indications to surgery. *Chemotherapy is also used for advanced cases.

Prevention of Cancer of the Cervix

Cancer of the cervix is one of the cancers that could be eliminated, using our current knowledge.

All women who are or ever have been sexually active should regularly undergo an examination of the cervix, and a *smear test. By the use of a *colposcope, the cervix can be scrutinized more thoroughly. This should be done annually until the menopause, unless it is advised otherwise. Thereafter a smear test every 3 years is adequate if previous tests have yielded normal results.

Abnormal cells in a smear test do not necessarily come from a cancer. Abnormalities caused by *papilloma virus infection develop within 2–3 years, but a smear test may not show abnormalities soon after infection even though the papilloma virus is present. Mild infection by other organisms in the vagina can cause abnormal cells in the smear.

If all sexually active women were screened regularly with *Pap smears and treated when abnormal cells were found, cervical cancer could be almost totally prevented.

The risk of cervical cancer can be reduced further by not *smoking, possibly by not using *oral contraceptives over many years, and by having only 1 sexual partner. Although the evidence is not conclusive, there are compelling reasons for each and every individual to take a good *diet. There is some evidence that a diet that protects against bowel and other cancers, that is, one containing adequate *vitamin A and avoiding other dietary deficiencies, will also protect against cervical cancer.

cesium-134 radioactive element having a *half-life of 2.06 years, released by nuclear reactors

cesium-137 radioactive element having a *half-life of 30.2 years. Cesium-137 is used in radiotherapy, replacing *radium and is released by nuclear reactors, as in the *Windscale and *Chernobyl accidents. See *atomic bombs and nuclear reactors.

CHEMICALS AS CAUSES OF CANCER

In 1775, Percivall *Pott, an English physician, first recognised the association between cancer of the *scrotum, a condition found in chimney sweeps, and *soot, which therefore became the first known chemical *carcinogen.

Soot consists of very fine particles of coal dust held together by *tar. One hundred years after Pott, the German surgeon *Volkmann recognized tar as the active carcinogenic agent in soot. In 1911 the Japanese researchers *Yamagiwa and *Ichikawa showed that tar could cause cancers by painting tar on the ears of rabbits. Now the individual cancer-inducing chemical compounds in the tar have been identified.

Since the discovery by Yamagiwa and Ichikawa of a way of inducing cancers for study, countless mice have been sacrificed to the cause of understanding cancer. The magnitude of this sacrifice pales into insignificance in comparison with the greatest continuing experiment in carcinogenesis, which uses as humans as subjects. This experiment is, of course, the *tobacco experiment.

The main classes of chemical carcinogens are *aflatoxins, *aniline dyes, *aromatic amines, *asbestos, *chloromethyl ethers, *metals, *nitrosamines, *oestrogens, *polycyclic hydrocarbons and *organochlorines, including *chlorinated insecticides and *trihalomethanes. *Tobacco contains chemicals from many of these classes of chemical carcinogens.

Evidence that a chemical is a cause of cancer is obtained in several ways: from studies of human populations exposed to it, by showing that the chemical causes cancer in experimental animals and by laboratory studies on *cells. In the *Ames test, demonstration of the power of a cancer to cause *mutations in bacteria alerts us to the potential for causing cancer, but a positive Ames test does not prove that a chemical is a carcinogen in man. *Organochlorines and chemicals of other classes may cause cancer in animals, while the proof that they cause cancer in humans may be lacking. See *cancer-inducing chemicals in food.

Table 4: Chemical agents which may cause cancer in humans

Agent	Site (industry)
*Aflatoxin	Liver
*Alcohol	Mouth, oesophagus, liver
*Aniline dyes and *aromatic amines	Bladder, kidneys
*Arsenic	Lung, skin, liver (in vintners)
*Asbestos	Lung, pleura, larynx
*Benzene	Leukaemias
*Benzidine	Bladder (rubber and dye industry)
*Chloromethyl ethers including *bischloromethyl ether	Lung
*Tars	Various (energy production, distillation of coal)
*Diethylstilboestrol	Uterus, vagina
*Hardwood dusts	Nasal cavities (cabinet making, woodworking)
Medications	
*Drugs for chemotherapy	Blood-forming organs, lymph nodes
*Aspirin, phenacetin	Kidney
*Metals and metallic compounds	
*Cadmium	Bladder, prostate, lung
*Chromium	Lung (metal plating, pigments)
*Nickel	Lung, nasal cavities (in nickel smelters)
*Mineral oils	Skin (metal industry)
*Mustard gas	Chemical warfare
*Naphthylamine (alpha and beta)	Bladder (rubber and dye industry)
*Nitrosamines	Stomach, bowel
*Polycyclic hydrocarbons	Skin, diverse
*Shale oils	Skin (energy production)
*Vinyl chloride monomer	Liver, blood vessels, lung

Other chemicals suspected of causing cancer are discussed under *occupation and cancer.

chemoprevention prevention of cancer by taking medications that inhibit the development of cancer. *Tamoxifen and *retinoids have potential for use in this way. Animal studies show that retinoids are effective in preventing certain experimentally-induced cancers. Chemopreventive agents may work by blocking the chemical events initiated by a *carcinogen. See *breast cancer.

*Clinical trials are being carried out of the use of retinoids in persons who have lung disease caused by *asbestos and in heavy smokers to determine whether *mesothelioma and *lung cancer can be prevented.

CHEMOTHERAPY

The word 'chemotherapy' was first used for treatment with drugs that selectively poison tropical parasites, first developed by the great German medical scientist, Paul *Ehrlich, in the early part of the century.

Chemotherapeutic medications are really poisons which work by blocking vital chemical processes. Many antibiotics are highly selective poisons for bacteria, but are not toxic to humans. Penicillin is usually a perfect chemotherapeutic agent against susceptible bacteria, poisoning the invading microbes without causing side effects in the patient. The reason for this is that many of the chemical processes which take place inside a bacterium differ considerably from the chemical reactions that take place in human cells.

It has proved more difficult to find chemotherapeutic agents for the treatment of cancer than for the treatment of bacterial infections. While cancer cells are obviously different from normal human cells, the differences are often extremely subtle. The chemical reactions taking place in cancer cells differ very little from those in normal cells. Indeed, the reactions are frequently the same, but their timing is wrong, or they are exaggerated.

Although *arsenic compounds had been used to combat cancer as early as the eighteenth century, the first of the modern drugs used to fight cancer had its origin in *mustard gas. It was discovered in World War I that mustard gas caused shrinkage of lymphoid tissues. In World War II it was observed that mustard gas and similar chemicals could arrest malignant growths for a short time. After World War II a systematic search for anticancer compounds was begun by designing compounds that would interfere with chemical processes that are essential for cellular function.

In many cancers, the proportion of proliferating cells is high. Many chemotherapeutic drugs are aimed at processes that take place in cell division. Normal tissues that replace their cells frequently, such as the blood and bowel, are unavoidably damaged by such drugs.

Chemotherapy usually controls cancer rather than curing it. However, some cancers are actually cured by chemotherapy. These are the cancers which are most sensitive to anti-cancer drugs. Examples are cancers of the *testis and the *lymphoid tissues. In these cases, cells of the body's defence mechanisms are probably involved in a mopping up operation to rid the body of the last surviving cancer cells.

Some cancers are so insensitive to all known chemotherapeutic agents that they are often considered not worth treating with chemotherapy. *Malignant melanoma and the commonest forms of *lung cancer fall into this category.

Between the cancers which are curable by chemotherapy and those which are resistant lies a group in which chemotherapy is effective, but virtually never curative. Recurrent *breast cancer is in this category. This cancer often responds very well at first, but relapses always occur.

How can *adjuvant chemotherapy, that is chemotherapy given at the time of surgery to wipe out tiny foci of residual tumour, be expected to work if the same chemotherapy never cures the disease when it has recurred? If chemotherapy is given when the number of cancer cells left in the body is very small, there is a chance that none will survive. Chemotherapy works best if given before the cancer becomes large, or immediately after most of it has been removed.

Fear of Cancer Chemotherapy

Cancer chemotherapy arouses the worst fears in the minds of many patients. When chemotherapy is advised, it often signals that the cancer is no longer curable. Most patients know of symptoms that chemotherapy causes, and dread them.

It is important to realize that different regimes of chemotherapy are used for different types of cancer, so symptoms experienced by one patient need not trouble another. Patients who have correctly been advised to have chemotherapy for relief of symptoms are almost invariably grateful and are glad to exchange the symptoms for the relatively minor side effects of chemotherapy. Unfortunately they cannot know this until they have tried the treatment.

Chemotherapy is given as tablets, or as injections or infusions into veins or arteries over hours or days. Intravenous treatment is usually not painful. If pain is experienced the patient should bring it to notice, because the drugs can sometimes have an irritant effect on the vein and if the needle comes out any drug spilt may irritate the skin or tissues.

Small instruments that pump chemotherapeutic drugs slowly into veins can be worn by patients to enable continuous treatment over days or weeks. Such treatment is in use in some centres for secondary cancer of the large bowel affecting the liver.

Some centres use 'regional chemotherapy', delivered slowly over hours or days into an artery, in order to deliver a high dose to a part

Table 5: Commonly used chemotherapeutic agents

Name	Preparation		Major Side Effects	
		immediate	days-weeks	late
bleomycin	(Blenoxane)	I	f	r	lung damage
carmustine	(BCNU)	I	n	h	
chlorambucil	(Leukeran)	T	n*	h*	
cyclophosphamide	(Cytoxan)	I,T	n	h,b,m	bladder irritation
cytarabine	(Cytosar, araC)	I	n	b	
doxorubicin	(Adriamycin)	I	n,f,v	h,b	heart damage
daunomycin	(Rubidomycin)	I	n,f,v	h,b	heart damage
dacarbazine	(DTIC)	I	n,v	h,b,m	
5 fluorouracil	(5-FU)	I	n	h,b,m,d	
hydroxyurea	(Hydrea)	T	n*	h,b,m,d	
melphalan	(Alkeran)	T	n*	b	kidney damage
methotrexate	(Methotrexate)	I,T	n	b,m	
lomustine	(methyl CCNU)	T	n	b,m	
mitomycin	(Mitomycin C)	I	n	b,m	
mitoxantrone	(Novantrone)	I	n,v	h,b	heart irregularity
cisplatin	(cis-Platinum)	I	n,v	h,b	kidney damage, hearing loss
procarbazine	(Natulan)	C	n	h,m	
vinblastine	(Velban)	I	v	h,b	muscle pains, constipation, stomach ache
vincristine	(Oncovin)	I	v	h,b	numbness, tingling fingers, toes
etoposide	(VP16-213)	I	n,v	h,b	

SYMBOLS: I = injection, T = tablet, C = capsule, b = low blood counts, f = fever, h = hair loss, n = nausea,
r = rash, v = damage to vein if injection leaks, * = uncommon

61

of the body with a large cancer burden. This technique can sometimes cause a cancer to shrink enough to make *surgery possible.

Whenever the patient is well enough, chemotherapy is given on an outpatient basis in a clinic, in doctors' rooms or even at home.

Resistance to Chemotherapy

A number of common cancers may respond initially to chemotherapy, but more resistant tumours evolve for a variety of reasons. Chemotherapy may kill a vast number of cancer cells, but some usually escape, again for a variety of reasons. Drugs that destroy dividing cells may not kill resting cancer cells. If the blood supply to part of a tumour is poor, the dose of drug reaching some cancer cells may be too low to kill them. *Mutations occur rather frequently among cancer cells. Resistance is often due to cancer cells making *P-glycoprotein, a substance which acts in the cancer cell membrane to pump chemotherapeutic poisons out. Because this chemical pump can eliminate a range of chemotherapeutic medications, cells that are resistant to one agent because they have P-glycoproteins may be resistant to other agents.

The reason for relapses after initial success with cancer chemotherapy is the evolution of new populations of cancer cells from the resistant cells. Even if chemotherapy can eliminate all but 1 cancer cell in 100 million, the surviving cell can multiply and give rise to a tumour composed of chemotherapy-resistant cells. Variant cells that grow best in the presence of the medication survive and outgrow those which are more sensitive to the drug. This is evolution at work in cancer.

To beat this tendency for resistant cells to develop, chemotherapy regimes usually consist of several drugs given in cycles. Typically the patient will receive drugs for a week or two then have a rest interval of 2 or 3 weeks. The rest interval allows the normal tissues to recover.

When a tumour recurs, signalling resistance, the options are to increase the dose or to change the drugs. It may be possible in future to plan chemotherapy by testing cancer cells from the patient's tumour in the laboratory, thus showing in advance which chemotherapeutic agents are effective. Development of P-glycoprotein by tumour cells in the presence of a drug would indicate that they can resist the drug.

Success with chemotherapy is always limited by the susceptibility of normal tissues to damage. Often a dose of cell poison that would eradicate the cancer would also kill too many normal cells. Many strategies are used, and more are under development, to overcome this limitation. *Bone marrow, which is sensitive to chemotherapeutic medications, can be removed before these are given, stored during treatment and returned to the body afterwards (see *bone marrow transplantation). The white cell *growth factor *G-CSF shows great

Table 6: Hormones used in cancer treatment

Type/Medication	Main Side Effects
Oestrogens	
ethinyl oestradiol	uterine bleeding
stilboestrol	fluid retention
Progestins	
medroxyprogesterone acetate	fluid retention
Androgens	
fluoxymesterone	masculinizing effects — deepening of the voice, growth of facial hair, increased sexual desire
Cortisones	
prednisone	diabetes, thinning of bones, change in
prednisolone	distribution of body fat, thinning of
dexamethasone	skin and easy bruising, blood clotting,
hydrocortisone	proneness to infections, mood
cortisone acetate	changes, increased appetite
Hormone blockers	
aminoglutethimide	life-threatening loss of mineral and fluid balance unless taken with regular cortisone
tamoxifen	hot flushes, uterine bleeding

promise in countering the depression of white blood cells caused by chemotherapy.

Patients may find themselves lacking appetite and energy during treatment courses, but there is no general prohibition on activity. It may be advisable to have a light meal on the evening of intravenous treatment to allow the stomach to settle. Unless there are severe side effects, patients can usually continue their normal activities, including sexual relations.

*Cortisone-type medications, particularly prednisone and predniso-lone, are commonly used in a number of chemotherapeutic regimes. Cortisone belongs to a class of hormones which are essential for life. Drugs of this class have many side effects, mostly not permanent, and not serious if cortisone is taken in cycles. They may lift the mood temporarily and make sleep difficult, and there may be a temporary drop in mood when they are stopped. Sleeplessness can be treated with an approved sleeping tablet. Cortisone can bring on diabetes in persons who have the tendency to develop this condition. It causes weight gain and indigestion. Use over prolonged periods causes muscle wasting and thinning of bones.

Side Effects of Chemotherapy

The intensity of the symptoms caused by chemotherapy varies widely. Chemotherapy causes lack of appetite and sometimes nausea. The symptoms are intensified by fear, anxiety and depression.

The right of patients to know of the side effects of their treatment poses the problem that a detailed description of all possible side effects can arouse unbearable fears. Doctors skilled in treating patients with cancer are acutely aware of the possibility of side effects. Their job is to get the best result with the fewest side effects. Patients have to enter into chemotherapy with the faith that their doctor is steering the best course between success and side effects.

As most drugs used in cancer chemotherapy affect dividing cells, the unwanted effects are seen in rapidly dividing blood forming cells and cells of the bowel and hair follicles of the scalp. Hearing, kidneys, bladder and other organs can be affected. The effect of chemotherapy on blood forming cells can cause low blood counts of (1) white cells and consequent susceptibility to infections, (2) *platelets, with risk of bleeding and (3) red cells, with *anaemia. These effects are the concern of the doctor administering the treatment, who will perform regular blood tests and other necessary checks for early signs of complications, before the patient experiences symptoms.

Because of lowered resistance to infection during chemotherapy, patients should should avoid people with colds or other severe infections. As chemotherapy may suppress early symptoms of infection, they should to seek advice when they feel generally unwell, even if the symptoms are mild.

Because many drugs may interfere with chemotherapy, medications such as vitamins, aspirin or pain-relieving drugs should not be taken unless approved or prescribed by the doctor. *Shingles is a painful rash which blisters, occurring with increased frequency in patients who receive chemotherapy. It is important to diagnose this condition early, preferably at the stage when the pain has started but the rash has not yet appeared, so that treatment with *acyclovir can be instituted.

Loss of hair   (*alopecia) is one of the most dreaded side-effects of chemotherapy. Although this is often not so severe as feared and the hair always grows back, the anticipation of loss of hair, then the loss of self-image when it occurs, may have a very serious psychological impact. Men may be affected just as badly as women. Some people readily accept the need to use a wig, others find the thought abhorrent. Patients on low incomes may be able to obtain a wig through Federal or State Government programmes, or through their State *Anti-cancer Society.

Hair consists of compacted dead cells, so no treatment of the hair itself will affect the outcome of chemotherapy. Hair is formed in follicles, pits in the skin, by cells which grow at the base of the follicle and die into it. Each hair follicle grows actively for 2 to 6 years, then rests. Ninety per cent of follicles are growing at any time. Growing cells in the active follicles are sensitive to a number of commonly used chemotherapeutic medications and loss of hair may begin from 2 weeks to 3 months after treatment is started.

The blood supply to the scalp can be interrupted temporarily by a tourniquet while medication is injected, to shield the follicles while the level of chemotherapeutic agent is high. Cooling of the scalp with ice packs has the same effect. These measures cannot be used when the patient is taking tablets, because drugs taken by mouth usually act over a long period.

A full head of hair may regrow within as little as 3–4 months, although it may take between 6 and 12 months after the end of treatment.

Oral Hygiene, Dental Caries and Chemotherapy

Ulceration in the mouth can be a problem with a number of medications used in chemotherapy. This problem usually resolves after treatment has stopped and can be helped by mouth washes and anti-microbial preparations if necessary. Oral *thrush is a problem, particularly if chemotherapy regimes contain *cortisone-type agents. Thrush responds to treatment with specific medications.

Dental hygiene is essential. Patients should see a dentist early, for attention to carious teeth and problems with gums. Preventive measures avert oral problems and preserve teeth.

Fertility, Infertility and Pregnancy

Women receiving chemotherapy should avoid becoming pregnant because anti-cancer medication can reach the developing baby. Patients who are taking birth control pills should discuss this with their doctors, because these can affect some forms of cancer, particularly *breast cancer.

Chemotherapy can stop menstrual periods and sexual drive could be decreased during the course of some types of treatment, depending on the general state of health.

*Infertility, often temporary, can arise from chemotherapy. Sperm counts may drop in men. Permanent infertility can arise in both men and women, but sperm counts rise or periods return in the majority of cases. See *testis cancer.

Commencement and Termination of Chemotherapy

Chemotherapy can only commence when patients have been given all reasonable information about the advantages and disadvantages of the treatment as it affects them. The doctor gives advice, and the patient decides. The patient is never under any compulsion to accept medical advice.

Chernobyl

Most physicians administer chemotherapy under the express condition that they may decide when it is in the patient's best interest to stop that treatment. Termination of the treatment may cause great anxiety to the patient because it may be seen as a sign of a deterioration of his or her condition. It is best if the patient knows of this possibility before treatment commences.

Conversely, every patient has the right to withdraw from treatment at any time after it has commenced. Patients should enter into chemotherapy with the understanding that they may exercise this right at any time.

Chernobyl Ukrainian city where meltdown of a nuclear reactor on 26 April 1986 led to a considerable fallout of radioactive substances in the Ukraine, Poland, the middle of Sweden and Finland, southern Bavaria and parts of Austria and Italy: regions housing a population of at least 5 million people. The most important exposure of the people was through the foodchains. In May 1986, many places had a high rainfall, which led to incorporation of radioactive substances into vegetable life, particularly grass. Radioactivity was seen early in milk, then in cereals, milk and meat during the next year. The main radioactive elements released in the accident were *iodine-131, *iodine-132. *cesium-134 and *cesium-137. See *atomic bombs and nuclear reactors.

childhood cancer Cancer affects only about 1 child in 8–900 before 15 years of age. However, cancer kills about as many children as do accidents. The incidence of childhood cancer in Queensland has apparently increased in the past 15 years to 1 in 500, according to figures of the Queensland Childhood Malignancy Register. This incidence is one of highest in the world when compared with other white-skinned populations.

The types of cancer occurring in childhood are mostly different from those occurring in adult life. This appears to be the result of different causative factors. In adulthood, environmental influences are thought to cause a large proportion of cancers. Environmental influences are probably much less important in causing childhood cancers. However, there is some evidence that breast feeding for more than 6 months protects against childhood cancer. *Heredity appears to be important and *viruses are suspected to be cofactors.

One third of childhood cancers are *leukaemias, one quarter are tumours of the brain and nervous system and one tenth are *lymphomas. Three other important types of childhood cancer are *Wilms' tumour *bone cancer and *retinoblastoma.

The most common childhood cancer is acute lymphoblastic *leukaemia. This used to be fatal in almost all cases. With dramatic improvements in treatment the condition can now be cured in the majority of children. See *leukaemia.

chlorambucil   drug used in *chemotherapy

chlordane   *chlorinated insecticide

chlorinated insecticides ('organochlorines')   These *organochlorine compounds are widely distributed in sprays, dusts, and solutions used as insecticides, despite legislation strictly limiting their use. In this class are DDT, aldrin, chlordane, dieldrin, endrin, heptachlor and lindane. Most of these cause acute toxicity, but the real concern is that animal experiments have shown chemicals of this class to cause cancer-like nodules in the liver. There is considerable controversy about the cancer risk from these substances. Cattle grazing on ground sprayed with these chemicals have detectable residues in their fat and the same applies to poultry reared in contaminated surroundings. The contamination may persist for decades and the chemicals in the food are taken up by the person eating the meat.

The insecticide DDT, a weak but definite carcinogen in animal tests, is almost impossible to avoid. DDT has spread over the globe, is concentrated in the fat of birds and mammals, and is in the plankton eaten by fish. At one stage Americans had 10 parts per million of DDT in their body fat—a level that would not be condoned in human food. A by-product of DDT, DDE, is detectable (1988 information) in virtually all samples of human milk in Australia in a concentration of about 20 parts per billion, about the same level as found in 1985.

Heptachlor and chlordane, two chlorinated insecticides that are made in USA, but not used there because of pressure by environmentalists, are used extensively in Australian households for the control of termites. The Australian problem is an abundance and range of termites, forcing a compromise between economic cost and health risk. One application of a chlorinated insecticide may protect the woodwork of a house for 30 years, illustrating both the advantage offered and the longevity which makes these compounds so risky.

Termite infestations can be avoided if a physical barrier is placed on the ground below a house. Other types of pesticides could be used which would confer no more than 5 years' protection after an application. There alternatives are much more expensive, at least to the houseowner.

chlorine   gaseous element with pungent odour which is very poisonous to humans in the free state. Chlorine is chemically highly reactive and forms *organochlorines with various animal and vegetable substances. See *water.

chloroform   chemical of the class of substances called *trihalomethanes, which may cause tumour nodules in the livers of mice. Chloroform was introduced in 1847 as a general anaesthetic agent, but is no longer in use for this purpose. Chloroform and other trihalomethanes develop during chlorination of *water.

chloromethyl ethers   class of carcinogenic chemicals, first used in the 1940s, including *bischloromethyl ether, a very powerful inducer of *lung cancer. The latent period, between exposure to chloromethyl ethers and the development of lung cancer, was shown in a study of of 737 American workers exposed to the chemical, to be 10–19 years.

chondrosarcoma   type of *bone cancer

choriocarcinoma   cancer of the *placenta

chromium   metallic element, which may cause cancer, and compounds of which may cause cancer. See *metals.

chromosomes   long paired threads of *DNA that correspond to chapters in the *genome. Chromosomes are strings of *genes. Each human cell contains 23 pairs of chromosomes, making up the genomic book or hereditary blueprint. See *gene, *genome, *nature of cancer.

chrysotile   white *asbestos

CIN, cervical intraepithelial neoplasia   a system of grading the premalignant and malignant changes in *smear tests for *cervix cancer. CIN I = moderate *dysplasia, CIN II = severe dysplasia and CIN III = definite cancer in situ (early cancer).

circumcision   cutting off the foreskin. Where hygiene is poor, circumcision reduces the incidence of cancer of the *penis.

cisplatin   medication used in cancer *chemotherapy.

clinical trial   study to test any new method or agent in medicine, conducted with the rigorous provisions necessary to obtain valid results. Such provisions are necessary to avoid the error of concluding that any benefit was actually due to the new method, when a better study would have shown that the difference apparently demonstrated by the trial was actually due to chance.

In order to obtain results that are not misleading, clinical trials must be large enough to give answers that are statistically valid. They must also avoid bias of all sorts. There are many ways in which a trial can be biased. Bias can be introduced if the person assessing the result knows what treatment the patient is receiving, or if the doctor conveys more confidence in one agent than another.

In the best clinical trials, the two types of treatment are compared prospectively, that is by starting the trial before the treatment is commenced, when nobody can guess the outcome, as distinct from beginning the comparison when the treatment is over. Retrospective trials can suffer from bias, by selecting patients that have done well under a particular treatment. The assessors should not know which treatment each patient has received. Another way of avoiding bias is to assign patients randomly, that is by a lottery over which the doctors have no control, to treatment A or treatment B, the two treatments which are being compared.

Clinical trials are regulated very strictly by the medical centres in which they are conducted. All plans for starting trials must be submitted to the Ethics Committee of the institution concerned. National bodies that support research using clinical trials are obliged to confirm that the appropriate Ethics Committee has approved the trial. The conditions must be explained fully to every patient who consents to enter a trial, and no patient may be used in a trial who has not signed a form of consent which explains fully the potential side effects and implications to him or her of entering the trial.

To the patient, a request to consider entering a trial may be very disturbing. The obvious questions are: Why does the doctor not know what is the best treatment? Why does he have to test the treatment? Why am I to be a guinea pig? At a time when patients need confidence, they have to be told that the best available treatments are not good enough.

There is no satisfactory alternative to clinical trials. All the preliminary studies in animals do not remove the need to study new treatments in humans before they can be used routinely. Many clinical trials are conducted internationally, recruiting patients from centres around the Western world and they involve huge expense. They are the guarantee to present and future patients of the validity of treatments and they are an instrument ensuring progress in the treatment of cancer. As a result of clinical trials, cancer treatment has changed beyond recognition from the state of the art 25 years ago.

The final note to patients who are asked to engage in clinical trials is: entry is purely voluntary; unless patients are completely satisfied, they need not be involved and should not be disadvantaged.

clone family of cells descended from one ancestor. All cells in a clone have the same genetic blueprint or *DNA.

coal tars source of cancer-inducing chemicals. See *chemicals as causes of cancer.

cobalt metallic element. Radioactive cobalt is used as a source of high-energy X-rays for *radiotherapy.

cocoa see *caffeine

codon   group of three of the basic units or letters of the *genetic code, forming a word of the code. See *gene, *genome.

coeliac disease   disease of the small bowel, causing diarrhoea and poor absorption of foods. Coeliac disease is due to sensitivity to the gluten fraction of wheat and the treatment is avoidance of all gluten in the food for life. Subjects with coeliac disease have a tendency to develop *lymphomas in the small bowel and they also have an increased risk of cancers of the *mouth and *oesophagus. The reason for these tendencies is unknown, but they are reduced by adhering to a gluten-free diet. See *heredity and cancer.

coffee   beverage suspected of playing a part in causing a number of cancers. As a result, many studies have been carried out to examine the possibility. One study showed a possible connection with *bladder cancer when 40 or more cups were drunk per week, but there is no good evidence that coffee itself causes cancer. The *caffeine in coffee also appears to be free of cancer risks. Many who drink a lot of coffee also smoke a lot, risking the dangers of *tobacco.

colon   the large bowel. See *bowel cancer.

colonoscope   long flexible *endoscope for examining the inside of the colon.

colonoscopy   examination of the bowel through a colonoscope.

colostomy   opening made surgically between the colon and the surface of the abdomen. A colostomy may be temporary, to enable the bowel to heal after a surgical procedure, or permanent, if a natural connection to the exterior cannot be preserved. Patients who have a permanent colostomy wear a special disposable appliance to collect faeces. They must be trained to manage the colostomy so that they can live with minimal restrictions necessitated by the condition. The opening of the colostomy, called the *stoma, needs to be cared for. Addresses of colostomy societies or associations in capital cities can be obtained from *Anti-cancer Societies.

colposcope   telescopic instrument for examination of the cervix of the uterus. See *cervix cancer.

computed tomography (CT)   type of X-ray examination permitting detailed views of different parts of the body, often revealing tumours not seen on conventional X-ray studies.

COPING WITH CANCER
When the diagnosis of cancer is made, there are three possible outcomes:

(1)   There is a very high chance of cure.
(2)   There is a chance of cure.
(3)   Cure is not possible.

The word 'cancer' generally summons up the third possibility, but this book is devoted to a positive attitude to cancer. Those who have not been able to avoid cancer may still have a good chance of cure, particularly with early treatment.

For those who cannot be cured, much can be done. New methods of treatment have become available in recent years, and new ways of defeating cancer are on the way.

Advice to Patients

If a cancer has been found and you are told that there is a very high chance of cure, you need only to make arrangements for treatment without delay.

If you have been found to have a cancer that has spread, and cannot be given a guarantee of cure, you will, without doubt, suffer great anxiety. Coping with the shock from the threat to health and life is difficult for anybody who finds he or she has cancer. Your doctor can give reassurance, but no immediate guarantee.

Pause for a moment, and consider a man who had a heart attack 7 years ago. He subsequently had a coronary bypass graft operation to relieve a blockage to a critical artery in the heart. This man is taking a very special holiday every year now, because he has no idea how long his reprieve will last. He knows he is not cured. He could have a heart attack at any moment. 'Every day is a bonus,' he says. **Every cancer patient who has had a reprieve is in the same situation.**

Most patients also ask the question: 'why me?' Working with cancer patients constantly reminds doctors that life is a lottery and that they too should cherish every day.

People who receive the news that they have incurable cancer need advice of a special kind.

The diagnosis of cancer strikes fear not only into the hearts of patients, but also into those of the family. To the patient, cancer has an impact that is different from the impact of any other disease. This impact is a mixture of shock, fear, dread, loathing, anger, depression, anxiety and often helplessness.

How can a person cope, having been told that he or she has cancer? If only he or she can overcome the impact and think clearly, but the emotions take over and crowd out all rational thought.

Here are some suggestions that may enable you to do the best for yourself.

Firstly, get the best medical advice.

Secondly, get independent confirmatory advice, unless it seems absolutely clear that you are in the hands of the best specialist or team of specialists.

Coping with cancer

Thirdly, understanding never did any harm and usually helps. This book aims to tell you what cancer is and does. It will not frighten you to know. On the contrary, understanding often counters fear.

If possible, take along somebody close to you when you go to the doctor. Most people will want to take their spouses. In many cases, a friend is the right person, and this is the time you need this friend.

When the doctor tells you about the cancer, your mind will be in a state of shock. In this state, your powers of concentration are greatly disturbed. While some aspects of the interview will be indelibly impressed upon your mind, others, which are equally important, will be forgotten completely. You are likely to misconstrue or misunderstand important things your doctor says, because your mind will be dwelling on other aspects of the interview.

When you have left the doctor, you should then go over the interview with the person who accompanied you. You must prepare the questions you will put at the next visit.

The question 'why me?' keeps coming back. People often have feelings of gross injustice. It is very likely that you will feel you have not deserved to be dealt with in this way. There is a point of view that people bring cancer upon themselves. This may be true in the case of those cancers caused by smoking or possibly by other recognized agents. Mostly, however, feelings of guilt are entirely out of place and uncalled for.

Everybody must have a personal philosophy to go through life and deal with its insults. No circumstance is likely to demand the use of your personal philosophy more, or to test it more, than finding out that you have cancer. If this philosophy, or personal rule book, has been left in a dusty cupboard or if the pages are blank where you are now looking, you will have to get a substitute, quickly.

Cancer is just one of the penalties in life's lottery and if you never thought about the lottery of life before, it would help if you did now. Remember that you have not finished with the lottery and you will get more surprises, not all of them bad.

Here is an essential thought about cancer, one that most people overlook. Cancer is but one of the diseases that strike mankind, and **it is not the worst.** Without doubt, it strikes as much fear as any disease can into the hearts of those affected, but just consider for one moment if the diagnosis had been something else.

Somehow or other, having to come to terms with heart disease seems quite different. 'Just a bit of trouble with the old ticker,' the patient will say, and friends will accept that. Heart disease has a respectability that cancer does not have. Many diseases strike worse blows (sudden death or paralysis are examples). But tell your friends it is cancer and their attitude will be different.

In fact, dealing with friends and relatives may at times seems the hardest part of dealing with the diagnosis of cancer. Friends often do not understand and they have the same mindless dread and incapacity to deal with cancer that the patient has when he or she first finds out.

The essential point is that cancer is not half as bad as many diseases we accept with much greater equanimity. It is better to have years of good life with cancer that a wretched short life with heart disease.

High blood pressure is another example. The patient comes away from the doctor, after receiving the news about high blood pressure, a bit bemused, thinking it is a bit of a nuisance, that one will have to think a few things through and make some changes in one's way of life. But it won't be too bad, one will carry on, there is no need to be too depressed about it.

In fact, with high blood pressure, there are risks of stroke, heart and kidney disease, and the tablets will have side effects. It is undoubtedly worse to have high blood pressure than some cancers.

Diabetes is another serious disease that does not engender the same fear as cancer. 'Just a bit of sugar,' the patient tells his family and friends. Diabetes, like high blood pressure, is usually not curable, but is well controlled by medical treatment. However, there are many bad complications of diabetes, and some diabetics will get these. That is their luck.

So, in many cases cancer has the same implications for the patient as high blood pressure, diabetes and heart disease, none of which can be cured. They have complications that shorten life, but life can be full and enjoyable if the maladies are properly controlled. Like cancer, each of these diseases can be fatal at any time. Many patients with heart disease, high blood pressure, diabetes, and many other diseases, would change places with various cancer patients, because their lot is far worse.

Reactions to being told of the diagnosis of cancer vary widely. A deep apathy may strike. Patients may be very angry with the world. There will be desperate concern for one's partner. There may be a frenzied desire to do something, anything, snatch at any straw, find the miracle that the doctors will not offer.

Patients often receive well-meant advice from friends. Frequently this advice is at variance with that given by the patient's own doctor, a very disturbing circumstance. This situation merits some thought. Who is likely to know best, the doctor who has devoted his life to your problem or the friend who knows what another friend found out from who knows where? You can always ask your doctor about this advice before taking any step.

The hardest thing is to think rationally. But you must.

You do not know how many years or months you may have, so, like the patients with incurable heart disease, high blood pressure or diabetes, you must get the best out of your life. You cannot afford to let your fears, depressions, anger and emotional turmoil rob you of daily pleasures.

Coping with cancer

You must reach a degree of acceptance that allows you to plan ahead, get as much fun in each day as you can, do the things you regard as important, and take your chances.

Remember back to the time before you had this sentence of cancer. You, like almost everybody else, probably did not think anything was going to happen to you. It is natural to deny the obvious (that is, that something bad is going to happen sooner or later). We all behave as if we are immune to life's dangers. When those imaginary guarantees are taken away, we desperately want them back.

In one respect, therefore, you now know better than most. You know how precious life is and you know that it is governed by chance. You have to see things more clearly than before, or you now have to rethink the things you, like the rest of us, have been ignoring all these years. You have to change your life to achieve the things that really matter, the important things. You have to do those each day, saying only 'I'm still here and I have another chance to do something important.'

What is most important to you is only known by you. It may be seeing your family, telling them you love them, doing something for somebody, looking at your favourite pictures, writing a letter, revisiting important places, making a long-deferred journey, drinking a fine wine, playing bridge with dear friends and so on.

You may have to make decisions about working, about finance, and about your assets.

But you may ask whether you can beat this thing by your own efforts. Many patients adopt the attitude that they are going to beat it, and that is helpful. What can the individual do personally, besides what the doctors are doing?

Will diet help? Will meditation help? Can the mind influence those marauding cancer cells? Do special exercises help? What about treatments that the medical profession won't use, won't even tell you about? See *alternative cancer treatments.

For many, religion is the key to understanding and coping. Diet, meditation, exercise and rest will all help. If they make you fell well, they are good. You must allow your body to do its best. Don't forsake your doctor if he or she advises you not to abandon othodox treatment in favour of an untried wonder cure. Don't forget that your doctor's reputation is on the line all the time. If you are not offered treatment that would give you a better chance, he or she is in trouble in more ways than one. Patients will tell others, other doctors will soon know and your doctor may even be sued. His livelihood depends upon giving you your best chances.

You need a doctor you can trust, one who will see you when you need him or her, one who will answer your questions. If yours does not meet with these standards, get another. It is your life and your feelings are more important than your doctor's.

In all this you may spare a thought for the doctors who have responsibility for cancer patients. They also have stresses. They like to win every case and they find it depressing when the enemy beats them. That is why they have to have holidays, have a break from this intensely demanding work. Therefore you will not be able to have one doctor who is always available to you. Most cancer doctors work in teams. From the point of view of the patient, this means that there is somebody who can deal with your problem at any time. Above all, the reputation of your doctor depends on the way he treats you. He cannot possibly risk denying you any kind of treatment that would benefit you.

Most English-speaking countries have cancer or *Anti-cancer Societies, devoted to the fight against cancer. As well as raising funds for research into cancer these societies provide various services and advice for cancer patients. For example, most have mastectomy, colostomy and laryngectomy support groups and they have a telephone 'hot line' for receiving calls by patients for advice and support.

copper sulphate   chemical added to water supplies to reduce growth of algae. Not known to cause cancer.

cortisone   *hormone produced by the adrenal gland, essential for life, exerting control on many body functions, including water and mineral balance, resistance to stress, use of body fats and sugar, and blood clotting. See *chemotherapy, *aminoglutethimide, *pain.

cosmic rays   *radiation of subatomic particles from outer space contributing to the unavoidable or background radiation.

cost of cancer   The emotional and social costs of cancer are incalculable. By making some very conservative assumptions, such as an average weekly income of just $100, it has been calculated that for each 1,000 who die, the loss of earnings would be over $30 million in the remainder of their working lives, not allowing for inflation. This is an enormous economic loss.

There are no good estimates of the cost of providing medical services for cancer patients. Reduction in the incidence of cancer would significantly reduce the burden of health services on the community, as cancer services are expensive. The annual cost in Australia of treatment of *skin cancers alone (other than *melanomas) has been estimated to exceed $A100 million.

cottontail rabbit papilloma virus   wart virus that causes cancerous warts in domestic rabbits, but not in wild rabbits. See *viruses and cancer.

creosote compound derived from coal or wood *tar, used in wood preservation. Repeated exposures may cause cancer of the *skin. See *occupation and cancer.

crocidolite blue *asbestos, a cause of *lung cancer and *mesothelioma.

Crohn, Burrill B 1884–1983, American physician, who described a disease of the bowel which he called regional enteritis, now known as *Crohn's disease

Crohn's disease type of chronic inflammation of the bowel, in which cancers may develop. Crohn's disease affects the small bowel more than the large bowel. There is an increased tendency for cancer to develop in both large and small bowels at sites where Crohn's disease affects the bowel.

cryolite mineral rich in *fluoride, also containing sodium and aluminium

cryotherapy treatment by freezing

CT scan see *computed tomography

cure of cancer Disappearance of all detectable traces of cancer tissue, as a result of treatment, is described as a *remission. It is usual to define 'cure' as maintenance of the cancer-free state for a definite time, for example five years. Patients with a 5-year 'cure' are unlikely to have recurrence of their cancer, but it is not rare for seedlings of some types of cancer to grow and become detectable after that time.

Curie, Pierre 1859–1906, and **Curie, Marie** 1867–1934, French physicists who isolated *radium from pitchblend in 1898. Marie Curie died of *leukaemia.

cyclophosphamide medication used in cancer *chemotherapy

cystoscope an *endoscope for examination of the bladder, introduced through the *urethra

cytarabine medication used in cancer *chemotherapy

cytology microscopic examination of *cells in tissue fluids, for example sputum and smears of the uterine cervix, for the detection of cancer cells and precancerous changes. Usually the diagnosis of cancer must be confirmed by microscopic examination of sections of tissue obtained by *biopsy.

cytomegalovirus widely distributed *virus usually causing minor illness with fever, but having severe effects on many unborn children. In *AIDS sufferers cytomegalovirus causes cancers.

cytoplasm part of *cells between the *nucleus and the cell's outer membrane. The cytoplasm is a liquid loaded with small organelles, *proteins (including *enzymes) in solution and fine fibres forming the cell's skeleton. Chemical processes essential for daily life take place in the cytoplasm.

Cytosar trade name of cytarabine, medication used in cancer *chemotherapy

Cytoxan trade name of cyclophosphamide, medication used in cancer *chemotherapy

D

2,4-D *organochlorine herbicide, component of *Agent Orange

dacarbazine medication used in cancer *chemotherapy

daminozide compound used to improve growth and colour of apples. See *cancer-inducing chemicals in food

daunomycin medication used in cancer *chemotherapy

DDE *chlorinated insecticide

DDT *chlorinated insecticide

deoxyribonucleic acid see *DNA

dermis layer of tissue underneath the *epidermis

diagnosis of cancer Various symptoms and signs observed by the examinig doctor point to the diagnosis of cancer. X-ray examination, scans and blood tests determine the site of cancer and the extent of spread. Some cancers release products that can be picked up in blood tests. However, it is essential in almost all cases to make the definite diagnosis by microscopic examination of a stained section of tissue obtained by *biopsy. The diagnosis can be missed if tissues removed at operation are not examined under the microscope. Conversely, a patient may be falsely judged to have cancer on appearances at operation if the tissues are not examined microscopically.

Modern methods of staining biopsied tissues have made the microscopic diagnosis of cancer a precise science, which permits the physician or surgeon to choose appropriate treatment and predict the outcome. Measurement of cancer products in the blood may, in some cancers of the *testis, *liver and *placenta show response to treatment and predict regrowth of tumours.

dieldrin *chlorinated insecticide

DIET AND CANCER
There seems no doubt that the food pattern in Western countries increases the risk of certain kinds of cancer. Diet is the likely explanation of the increased incidence of cancers of *breast, *ovary, *bowel,

78

*uterus and *prostate in migrants from countries like Japan, where the risk is low, to countries like America where the risk is high. Also the falling incidence of *stomach cancer is most probably related to subtle changes in what we eat.

Animal evidence confirms that diet as a risk factor in the causation of cancer. The cancer rate in experimental animals is significantly reduced by underfeeding them.

One of the greatest epidemiologists, Sir Richard *Doll, considers that the evidence against *obesity justifies public education. Simply overeating, if it leads to overweight, increases cancer risks. Limitation of calorie intake sufficient to avoid obesity would certainly help reduce the risks of cancer of the *gall bladder and *uterus.

Lack of essential components, such as *vitamins, *minerals and *fibre, may be important in inducing cancer. *Fats (particularly animal fats), especially if intake is high, are suspected of being a factor in causing *bowel and *breast cancers. Other factors in the diet are contamination of food with cancer-causing *chemicals, such as *nitrosamines, *polycyclic hydrocarbons and possibly *pesticides. *Alcohol is a factor in development of cancer of the *mouth, *oesophagus and *liver and is now thought to increase the risk of breast cancer slightly.

There has been much concern that *food irradiation, which has great advantages in preventing decay and spoilage of food, may cause cancer. Present knowledge does not suggest that the risk is great, but there can be no certainty until sufficient experience has been gained.

A Recommended Dietary Pattern

The Dietitians Association of Australia has made the following dietary recommendations to reduce the risk of cancer:

1. Choose a varied and adequate diet to ensure that intake of known and unknown protective factors is more likely and that exposure to any known or unknown risk factors will be reduced.
2. Avoid excessive energy intake, aiming at a healthy body weight.
3. Control the amount of *fat and *protein in the diet, keeping added fats and oils down to a minimum, choosing lean meats and increasing consumption of cereals, beans, peas, lentils and legumes.
4. Eat liberal servings of dark green and yellow vegetables and fruit each day. Both *vitamin A and *carotenes in plant foods, from which vitamin A is made, appear to offer some protection against the risk of some forms of cancer. Vitamin A is toxic in large quantities and is not recommended as a regular supplement. The carotenes are not toxic and the regular use of fruit and vegetables

not only provides this vitamin but other valuable nutrients as well.

5. Every day, and preferably at each meal, eat fruits and vegetables such as citrus, berries, tomatoes and capsicums, all rich sources of *vitamin C and all capable of inhibiting the formation of carcinogenic *nitrosamines in the stomach.

Very large doses ("megadoses") of vitamin C are not recommended.

6. Include some dairy products in the daily diet. Several substances in milk foods, including vitamin D, have been suggested as protective against cancer. The use of low fat dairy foods will help keep the total intake of fat down.

7. Use in moderation foods cured or pickled with salt, *nitrates or smoke.

8. Avoid excessive consumption of alcohol.

Public Health Measures to Improve Diet

As about 35% of cancer is caused by faulty diet, how can this be addressed?

Cost of food is a major factor in determining diet in Western countries. Unfortunately fresh fruits and vegetables, and lean meats constitute more expensive choices than the undesirable high-fat, low-fibre foods.

So-called 'fast food' is immediately satisfying and has become socially acceptable. Much of it incorporates the high-fat, low-fibre choice.

Besides economic measures to enable the choice of good food, the diet of a society can be influenced by education and public opinion. We have made little progress in this respect. One index of the nutrition of a society is the proportion of obese people. Obesity is frequent in most Western countries.

Dietary advice needs a secure foundation. A campaign to change the diet of a nation should be based on solid evidence that what is advocated will be successful. Unfortunately, although the evidence incriminating bad diets in causing cancer is strong, because of the very clear differences between countries like Japan and USA (see *geographical distribution of cancer), it is much less clear what is wrong with these diets. As there are great differences in the fat, fish and animal meat contents of the diet of the two nations, we deduce that these are the cause of the differences in cancer incidence. However, we have not positively identified all the factors in American and Japanese diets that cause cancer, or what factors in these diets protect against the development of cancer.

There are compelling reasons to work for a change in the diet of Western nations, other than those relating to cancer. Diet also influences the development of heart disease and stroke, and the diets which help prevent these diseases are virtually the same as those which we believe will help reduce the cancer risk.

diet for cancer patients People who have cancer usually wonder whether dietary measures will help them in their fight.

While there is no convincing evidence that diet alone is effective as a treatment for cancer, nutritional care can play an important role in improving the quality of life for many people who have cancer.

All cancer patients should eat a good diet which provides the needed calories, *proteins, *fats, *carbohydrates, *minerals and *vitamins. Essentially this means good meat, vegetables and fruit.

There is no evidence that excessive intake of vitamins or minerals, honey, royal jelly or particular fad food can make any difference to the cancer, although patients may place great store by such regimes. The body simply does not use excessive doses of vitamins. There is no good evidence that any diet has a curative effect on cancer.

If there were the slightest evidence that a particular diet would reduce the growth of cancers, no cancer doctor would fail to tell his or her patients about it, simply because his or her reputation is at stake.

Fig. 14: Diet

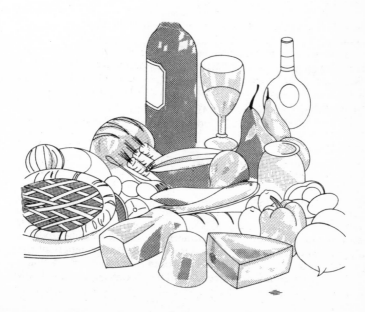

Diet therapy

Cancer patients can experience a range of difficulties with food intake. These problems often require the help of experts—dietitians and doctors—to maintain appropriate nourishment. Patients undergoing *radiotherapy or *chemotherapy often lose their appetites. Attention to diet often greatly helps these people come through their treatment. Sometimes nutritional support, by way of tube feeding, or intravenous feeding, may greatly help tolerance to treatments.

Patients with advanced cancer who are losing weight should be given a diet rich in sugar and carbohydrate, because they do not use sugar efficiently. This inefficiency is partly due to insulin not putting sugar into the cells and it can be overcome by taking in more sugar, unless the patient has diabetes.

Patients often ask about appetite stimulants. Perhaps the best is alcohol in moderation (if permitted by the doctor). A glass of whatever kind of alcoholic drink the patient fancies will often make the evening meal more enjoyable.

There are few other useful substances which can be used to improve appetite. Medications of the *cortisone class boost appetite, but are often not appropriate because they cause side effects.

diet therapy   see *alternative cancer treatments

diethylstilboestrol   medication of the *oestrogen class. This medication was formerly given to prevent miscarriages. Daughters of the treated women developed cancer of the *vagina, an otherwise very rare cancer.

diethyl sulphate   chemical suspected to cause cancer.

differentiation   process of maturation of *cells from immaturity to functional competence. See *nature of cancer

dimethyl-benzanthracene (DMBA)   chemical of the *polycyclic hydrocarbon class that can induce cancer. See *chemicals causing cancer.

dimethyl-aminoazobenzene (DAB)   *aniline dye that can cause cancer of the *bladder. See *chemicals causing cancer.

dimethyl sulphate   chemical compound used as a solvent, suspected to cause cancer

dioxins   subclass of *organochlorines. Tetrachlordibenzodioxin, TCDD, an ingredient of *Agent Orange, has been an important issue for two decades, during which it has been studied intensively. Paper-mill sludge is a major source of TCDD. Although much is known about these substances, how they act is still unclear. It appears that humans are much less sensitive to the acute effects of dioxins than some animal species and there is said to be no documented human death resulting from exposure to them.

Dioxin promotes cancer in experimental animals, but does not initiate it. This means that dioxin does not cause cancer by itself, but if given after a cancer-causing chemical, the animal is more likely to develop cancer. See *initiator, *promoter.

In 1976, an explosion in a plant near Seveso, Italy, caused contamination of a populated area by dioxin. A study in 1989 reported mortality greater than expected from a number of types of cancer and less for other types.

DNA, (*deoxyribonucleic acid*) is the substance that constitutes the hereditary material of almost all living creatures. (Some viruses use *RNA.) Each cell of an individual contains the same blueprint, written in DNA code, that controls its growth and behaviour. Besides blueprints for all human characteristics of height, hair colour, shape of face and so on, our DNA also makes each of us a unique individual, unless we have an identical twin.

The code for the information is beautifully simple. DNA is an extremely long set of instructions, written with only four chemical letters, also known as bases or nucleotides, referred to in shorthand as A, T, G and C. Each word uses only three of these letters. Each word stands for a particular *amino acid, a building block of *protein. The complete sentence (*gene) is the total instruction by which cells make a key class of substance, *protein. See *genetic code.

The string of letters making up DNA has a spiral or corkscrew shape and normally exists as a double spiral. In this double spiral, known as the *double helix, the letters or bases on one spiral are matched in a strict way with bases on the other spiral. A on one spiral always matches with T on the other, C with G, and conversely, T with A, G with C. This specific matching in the double helix provides a back-up copy of the *genes and is the basis for the exact copying of the DNA in a dividing cell. By splitting the spirals and matching the letters on each half spiral when it divides, a cell gives each daughter cell an exact copy of its DNA. This process is illustrated in Fig. 32.

Cancer results from particular types of alteration of a cell's DNA. See *gene, *genome, *chromosome, *nature of cancer.

Mapping of the whole of the human DNA has begun. By the end of the century, the sequence of letters in the DNA of a typical human will have been described by a world-wide organization known as Hugo, the Human Genome Organization. The sequence will occupy 200,000 pages of dictionary-size small print.

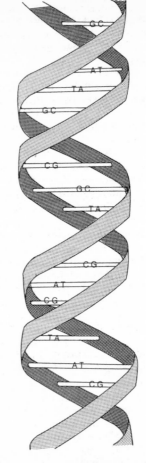

Fig. 15:

DNA, the double helix. The hereditary material, DNA, which encodes the characteristics of most living creatures, is basically a simple chemical structure. It usually exists as two long strands, like corkscrews. One is the master strand, which is used by the cell as the information storage. The other is a backup strand. Each spiral forms the backbone of the chemical structure. Protruding from the backbone like rungs of a ladder are the chemical letters of the genetic alphabet, designated A, T, G, and C. Each chemical letter on the master strand always matches with the complementary letter on the backup strand. A always matches with T and G always matches with C. This can be seen more simply when the spirals are untwisted, to give DNA the form of a ladder, as illustrated in Fig. 30.

Doll, Sir Richard contemporary cancer epidemiologist, formerly professor of medicine in Oxford. Doll's work provided proof of the relationship between *tobacco and cancer. He also contributed greatly to the epidemiology of *leukaemia and of carcinogens other than tobacco. See *asbestos, *diet, *tobacco.

double helix structure having two parallel spirals. *DNA has this structure. Hence, DNA is often referred to as the 'double helix'.

Down, John 1828–1896, London physician who described the syndrome that bears his name.

Down's syndrome condition formerly known as mongolism, caused by an abnormality of chromosomes (an extra chromosome) occurring in development of the unfertilized ovum, which predisposes to the development of a type of *leukaemia. See *heredity and cancer.

doxorubicin medication used in cancer *chemotherapy

drug addiction see *addiction

DTIC trade name of dacarbazine, medication used in *chemotherapy

dysplasia irregular growth of cells. See *cervix cancer.

dysplastic naevus syndrome condition predisposing to the development of *malignant melanoma. See *skin cancer.

E

Ehrlich, Paul 1854–1915, one of Germany's greatest medical scientists, professor in Berlin and Frankfurt and Nobel Prize winner in 1908, who pioneered chemotherapy of infectious microorganisms, and many other advances. As a medical student he made an enormous contribution to medicine by introducing staining of blood cells, fundamental to haematology. He also studied immunity in cancer, antibodies, infectious diseases and plant toxins.

electromagnetic radiation spectrum of radiation that includes visible light. Electromagnetic radiations from the sun include electric waves, radio waves, infrared rays, visible light, *ultraviolet light and *X-rays.

endoscope an instrument for examination of the interior of a hollow organ or body space

endrin *organochlorine insecticide

environment and cancer Two kinds of influence determine the occurrence of cancer, environment and *heredity. The environment acts on the body, and its hereditary constitution dictates the way environmental forces are dealt with.

The air, water and soil are the source of external influences on the body that can induce cancer. The individual can regulate his *diet and the drugs he takes, but is powerless to stop breathing polluted *air, drinking polluted *water, or eating contaminated food.

Every stretch of land on the globe and every body of water contains man-made chemical substances that were not present 100 years ago, such as *chlorinated insecticides and *polychlorinated biphenyls. These measurable pollutants are an indication that there are many more such widespread compounds.

Many *chemicals are recognized as causes of cancer. All of these can pollute a local environment. The extent of current pollution notwithstanding, less than 5% of cancers can be attributed to general pollution. The major concern must be the ongoing pollution in the increasingly industrialized planet.

The greatest driving force of pollution is the global population, which reached 5 billion in 1987. The Western nations contribute disproportionately to global pollution.

Governments have to face choices of unparalleled difficulty in balancing commercial needs, environmental degradation and pollution. As an example, the human requirement for vast amounts of paper results in the chemical treatment of logged trees, leading to release of *dioxin into the environment. The potential of these substances for widespread effects on animal and vegetable life, impinging on human food chains, is unknown. Consumers can reduce the chemical hazards associated with our consumption of paper by the use of unbleached and recycled paper wherever it is possible, and governments can adopt measures to encourage such usage.

Types of pollution are discussed under *air pollution, water, *chemicals causing cancer and *occupation and cancer.

enzyme type of *protein that facilitates chemical reactions in the body. Enzymes are the working tools of living matter for making all body constituents and providing the energy for life.

epidemiological studies Sir Richard *Doll has defined epidemiology as 'the study of the variation in the incidence of disease under the conditions of life experienced by different groups of people' (Reference Bannasch in Appendix). Epidemiological studies have been one of the most important forms of research into the causes of cancer.

Essentially, an epidemiological study compares two groups of people who are as similar as possible, except for one characteristic. For example, to determine the cancer risk of *tobacco smoking, the smoking and non-smoking groups should be as similar as possible with respect to age, sex, occupation, exposure to other known cancer risks etc., differing only in that the subjects in one group do not smoke.

Early epidemiological studies identified sexual activity as a factor in the causation of cancer of the *cervix; soot as a cause of cancer of the *scrotum in chimney sweeps; and *radiation in mines as a cause of *lung cancer.

As an example of the power of epidemiological studies in identifying causes of cancer, it has been demonstrated that although certain cancers are relatively common at certain sites in countries all over the world, the incidence of these common cancers varies considerably from place to place. Moreover, by choosing groups of the same race in different parts of the world, it has been shown that the differences in incidence are associated with the place, and factors in the lives of the people there, rather than their racial constitution. It is therefore considered that *heredity is much less important than *environment and *lifestyle in determining the incidence of common cancers.

The precision of epidemiological studies increases as it becomes possible to define more precisely the factors affecting different groups of people. The hazards in the environment, including the workplace, are established by precise measurements of known or suspected cancer-inducing agents in the surroundings and in the blood or urine of the subjects. Taking the early examples cited above, when knowledge increased it was possible to show that *papilloma virus was the factor associated with sexual activity in causation of cancer of the cervix; *radon was the factor causing lung cancer in miners; and *tar was the

87

factor in soot that caused cancer of the scrotum. In the latter case, the carcinogenic chemical agents in tar have been identified.

The principles of epidemiological studies and the techniques employed are essentially the same as those used in *clinical trials.

epidermis outermost layer of *cells in the skin

epithelium layer of cells lining body surfaces, for example, skin, mouth and bowel

Epstein-Barr virus (EBV) a virus occurring all over the globe. In countries with good sanitation and hygienic standards, the first infection with Epstein-Barr virus usually causes glandular fever (also known as infectious mononucleosis), commonly among students at the end of secondary education, frequently at examination time!

EBV can cause cancer in certain settings. It is a causative factor in *Burkitt's lymphoma, *nasopharyngeal carcinoma and cancers in patients with *AIDS. In countries where Burkitt's lymphoma is endemic, Epstein-Barr virus infects children in the first few years of life. See *viruses causing cancer.

erythropoietin a *growth factor produced in the kidneys, which is necessary for adequate production of red blood cells in the *bone marrow. *Anaemia due to poor bone marrow function is a serious problem in many chronic illnesses including cancer. Erythropoietin produced by gene technology has recently become available to treat persons whose kidneys do not produce enough. Erythropoietin may have a part to play in treatment of people who have become anaemic because of cancer chemotherapy.

etretinate *retinoid-type medication

Ewing, James 1866–1943, professor of pathology at Cornell University, New York, who described the cancer now known as *Ewing's sarcoma

Ewing's sarcoma a *bone cancer occurring in children and young adults

familial adenomatous polyposis (FAP) hereditary condition predisposing to *bowel cancer. Affected persons develop numerous *polyps
in the large bowel by the age of 20 and there is a high risk of
developing large bowel cancer in one or more of these by the late 30s
to mid 40s. Children of an affected person have a 50% chance of
developing FAP and offspring who do not inherit the responsible
*gene do not pass FAP onto their descendants. Males and females are
equally at risk and the disease does not skip generations. Although
inheritance of FAP can often be traced from generation to generation, in 10%–20% of cases the disease arises from a spontaneous
*mutation in a member of a family not previously affected by FAP.
Many countries have established registers of FAP families.

The condition is detected by examination of the lower bowel
through a *colonoscope. If annual investigation fails to detect polyps
by the mid-20s, subjects are regarded as being free of FAP. Persons
who have the condition need appropriate surgery. See *bowel cancer.

The abnormality in *DNA which leads to familial polyposis can
now be detected by *gene probing. The same abnormality occurs in
patients with no family history of bowel polyps or cancer, presumably
induced by an agent in food or in the environment.

fat Fat is one of the major classes of foodstuffs, along with *protein
and *carbohydrate. It is distinguished by its greasy nature, by not
dissolving in water and melting at low temperatures. A high content
of animal fats is probably an important factor causing cancer of the
large *bowel. The large bowel, in contrast to other parts of the body
which get all of their nourishment from the bloodstream, can use
some fats directly from the contents of the bowel for its own nutrition. An oversupply of certain types of fat in the bowel contents may
cause a growth disturbance of cells lining the bowel, promoting the
development of cancer cells.

A high intake of fat is also suspected of being a causative factor of
*breast cancer.

fibre Vegetable fibre is made of long chains of *carbohydrate. It
comes largely from the walls of plant cells, much of which is not
digested by humans. Animals do not make similar fibre and it is not
required for nutrition. The British doctor Dennis *Burkitt, noticed
that Africans have large stools but virtually no bowel cancer. The diet
of the Africans is also rich in certain vegetable fibres. These two
observations have suggested that fibre may protect against bowel
cancer. In the industrialized West the diet contains more animal fat,
more beef and more refined carbohydrate than the native African
diet.

Fibre may protect against cancer in a number of ways. It hastens
the passage of bowel contents, reducing the exposure to *carcinogens.

Fibreglass

The time for bacteria to produce carcinogens from fats is reduced and the increased bulk simply dilutes carcinogenic substances.

Research into dietary fibre is difficult because there are a number of types of fibre, which are hard to measure. Although the case for a protective effect of fibre is not watertight, a diet that contains a relatively high content of fibre is good for other reasons. Foods rich in fibre include most vegetables, particularly cereals and cereal products, fruits and nuts. A diet rich in sugars (including soft drinks), refined flour (biscuits), dairy products, meat and fats will be low in fibre.

fibreglass   material made with styrene resin and glass fibres. While there is no evidence relating styrenes to cancer, glass fibres can undoubtedly cause lung cancer if they are the right size to be inhaled. Fortunately, glass fibres in fibreglass are too big. A study of 4734 employees at an English glass fibre plant showed no significant risk of lung cancer. See *asbestos.

fluoride and cancer   Much alarm has been engendered by opponents of the addition of fluoride to *water supplies, who have blamed fluoride for causing cancer.

*Epidemiological studies have disproved these allegations. In English and American studies, no relationship has been shown between cancer mortality and the level of fluoride in water. One half of the population of the US, which does not have access to water with an optimal fluoride concentration of 1 mg per litre, has the same cancer rate as those drinking fluoridated water. Among *cryolite workers in Copenhagen, who had very heavy exposure to fluoride over many years, a small increase in lung cancers was found, but this association may not be significant because smoking by the workers was not taken into account.

Fluoridation in the US is also not associated with heart disease, diseases inside the skull, liver disease or *Down's syndrome. Fluoridation of water does not cause disfiguring dental fluorosis, hypersensitivity, fluorosis of bones, intolerance reactions or chronic poisoning.

5 fluorouracil   medication used in cancer *chemotherapy

fluoxymesterone   synthetic *hormone of the *androgen class used in treatment of *breast cancer. See *chemotherapy.

food irradiation   There is great debate about the potential of irradiated food to cause cancer. By killing all forms of life within food— bacterial, viral, animal (including insect) and vegetable, irradiation is a method of preservation that offers enormous economic advantages. Food need never go mouldy or become infested with weevils or other insects. Food poisoning, resulting from the overgrowth of bacteria that produce toxins, can be prevented.

One school of thought regards irradiation of food as simply another form of *electromagnetic radiation — like heat. Cooking also changes the molecules in food and certainly produces small amounts of *carcinogens, such as the *benzpyrenes. According to this point of view, irradiation is no worse than cooking. Furthermore, it is possible that food irradiation may reduce exposure to carcinogenic chemicals in food caused by microorganisms and insects.

The other point of view holds that irradiation damages *DNA molecules, as well as many other types of molecule, resulting in products which have the potential to cause cancer. There is animal evidence that seems to support this point of view, but there is a great deal of controversy about the validity of that evidence.

Irradiated food has been shown to contain rather high levels of free radicals, which are chemically reactive groups of atoms that can damage cells of the body. Again, free radicals are formed all the time in the body, so the danger depends on the type and quantity of free radicals consumed.

The World Health Organization and the United Nations Food and Agriculture Organization have made recommendations on food irradiation (see Appendix). So far, 33 countries have cleared irradiated food for human consumption and in many of those, its use is strictly limited.

It seems prudent to wait before more evidence is available to allow a proper judgment before the unregulated use of food irradiation is allowed. The costs of failing to resist the pressures to make profit from new but untested technology may be enormous. As an example, many deleterious aspects of the impact of motor vehicles may have been avoided by waiting while the evidence was gathered, before they were made in their millions.

formaldehyde   material with an acrid odour, used as bactericidal and embalming agent, the active constituent of *formalin, also used in medical, technology. As formaldehyde causes *mutations in certain bacteria and in human *cells in the test tube, it has the potential to cause cancer. Strict precautions should therefore be taken in handling formaldehyde, to prevent inhalation, ingestion or touching the skin.

formalin   preparation of *formaldehyde

foundries   factories where *metals and other materials are melted. Hot gases from steel and nickel foundries have been held to cause cancer of the *lung. Lung cancer mortality was increased among 4393 men employed in a zinc-lead-cadmium smelter, especially those employed for more than 20 years, but it was not possible to determine whether the risk was due to a particular element. Soil sampling in the districts surrounding foundries is used as proof of air pollution by metals. See *occupation and cancer.

G

gallbladder cancer The gallbladder lies under the liver beneath the ribs on the right side of the abdomen. Cancer of the gallbladder is uncommon. It may cause indigestion, grumbling abdominal pain or discomfort. Gallbladder cancer occurs in persons who have had gallstones for many years. It is not known whether chronic inflammation or irritation by the stones cause the cancer, or whether the disease that causes the stones is also a factor in causing the cancer.

*Surgery can cure only a quarter of cases of gallbladder cancer, because the condition is usually diagnosed late. *Radiotherapy may help, but *chemotherapy is not usually very helpful.

The chance of cancer developing in gallbladders containing stones is not great enough to warrant operation, but removal of the gallbladder is generally recommended to forestall attacks of inflammation of the gallbladder later in life.

Gallo, Robert contemporary American virologist, co-discoverer with *Montagnier of *human immunodeficiency virus (HIV)

gamma globulin fraction of blood that contains *antibodies. Human gamma globulin preparations are used to prevent infections in patients whose *immunity is defective.

gastroscope an *endoscope for viewing the inside of the stomcah

G-CSF and GM-CSF (granulocyte and granulocyte macrophage-colony stimulating factors, respectively), *growth factors for white blood cells. GM-CSF was used to treat damage to *bone marrow in *Chernobyl victims. G-CSF has been heralded as probably the single most important discovery in cancer *chemotherapy of the past few years. These substances reduce the danger of serious infection from a fall in white blood cell counts.

gender the sex of an individual. Gender is a major factor determining the development of cancer. Of course, cancers of the reproductive organs occur only in the males or females, but other types of cancer occur more frequently in one sex or another. For example, cancer of the *kidney occurs nearly twice as often in males as in females. Cancer of the *lung is much more common in males, but this is due to *tobacco smoking being predominantly a male habit, until recently.

gene unit of heredity, specifying inherited characteristics. A gene corresponds to a word in the *genetic code, containing the information for a cell to make a *protein. A string of genes makes up a *chromosome.

genetic code The whole genetic code is reproduced here, to show how simple it is and because the breaking of the code represents a magnificent achievement in man's understanding of life processes. Cancer results from falsification of the words or sentences, written in this code, in the cell's genetic blueprint.

Essentially, the DNA alphabet has four letters, A, C, G and T. Each word (technically known as a *codon) has three letters. A *transcript of a DNA sentence is made in the closely similar chemical letters of *RNA as a pattern for making the corresponding *protein. Three of the letters of RNA, namely A, C, and G are the same as the letters in DNA, but instead of T, RNA uses U.

The *translation of the DNA code is given in Table 7. Each three-letter word signifies an *amino acid, a building block of the cellular material called *protein. A set of words, ie a sentence, makes up a *gene. Protein is made by joining amino acids together in the order specified in the RNA transcript. The translation of an RNA transcript or message is illustrated in Fig. 33.

To find which amino acid building block is encoded by a word, look up the first letter, the second and then the third. For example, TAC corresponds to the amino acid Tyr, shorthand for tyrosine.

Table 7: The genetic code

1st letter	2nd letter				3rd letter	Amino acid	
	T	C	A	G			
T	Phe	Ser	Tyr	Cys	T	Ala	Alanine
T	Phe	Ser	Tyr	Cys	C	Arg	Arginine
T	Leu	Ser	STOP	STOP	A	Asn	Asparagine
T	Leu	Ser	STOP	Trp	G	Asp	Aspartic acid
						Cys	Cysteine
C	Leu	Pro	His	Arg	T	Glu	Glutamic acid
C	Leu	Pro	His	Arg	C	Gln	Glutamine
C	Leu	Pro	Gln	Arg	A	Gly	Glycine
C	Leu	Pro	Gln	Arg	G	His	Histidine
						Ile	Isoleucine
A	Ile	Thr	Asn	Ser	T	Leu	Leucine
A	Ile	Thr	Asn	Ser	C	Lys	Lysine
A	Ile	Thr	Lys	Arg	A	Met	Methionine
A	Met	Thr	Lys	Arg	G	Phe	Phenylalanine
						Pro	Proline
G	Val	Ala	Asp	Gly	T	Ser	Serine
G	Val	Ala	Asp	Gly	C	Thr	Threonine
G	Val	Ala	Glu	Gly	A	Trp	Tryptophane
G	Val	Ala	Glu	Gly	G	Tyr	Tyrosine
						Val	Valine

The amino acids are designated by three-letter symbols, which are defined in the right-hand column. For example, Lys signifies the amino acid lysine. The words UAA, UAG and UGA, decoded as STOP, occur at the end of a genetic sentence and function to terminate the translation.

This simple code has plenty of reserve for writing down all the information that is needed in the blueprint of any living creature. There is virtually no limit to the order of the building blocks in a protein and since there are hundreds of amino acids in the average protein, there is no limit to the number of distinct proteins that can be encoded.

Understanding the genetic code was a step towards *genetic engineering. The cracking of the genetic code represents a towering achievement of modern science, which makes it possible to reveal the true nature of cancer and which will, without doubt, lead to ways of defeating the disease.

genetic engineering The term 'genetic engineering', also called 're-combinant gene technology' or 'gene splicing', refers to the transfer of *genes, from one type of cell into another, or to the alteration of existing genes. Gene splicing conveys the image of inserting frames into a strip of motion picture film. When the film is screened, the new images become part of the whole. A scene from 'Gone with the Wind' could become part of 'Crocodile Dundee'. Using our comparison of the *genome with a book, genetic engineering is the insertion of words, sentences or even chapters.

It is interesting to compare and contrast *mutations and genetic engineering. Mutations are changes to DNA occurring by chance and are generally undesirable, Mutations caused by *radiation and various chemicals cause random damage to DNA, with unpredictable results. Genetic engineering is the deliberate creation of a mutation of a precise kind, for a defined purpose.

Evolution occurs by natural selection of favourable mutations. Genetic engineering achieves mutations favourable to the human genetic engineer's purposes. People have used selective breeding of plants and animals from prehistory. Genetic engineering to obtain bigger animals and better plants achieves the same result as selective breeding, but greatly reduces the time to do it.

By gene splicing, a substance normally made by one cell, for example human insulin, can be made in another cell, such as a bacterium. When a gene from one organism is inserted into a cell of another species, it is usual to add another gene that turns the new gene on. In this way, the new cell not only has the gene, but also uses it to make the desired product of the gene.

The consequences of being able to do this are, without exaggeration, revolutionary. The gene may come from any living creature and may be inserted into virtually any type of cell. Journalists use colourful phrases to describe the potential, such as 'organisms made to order'. They ask if genetic engineering is a mighty step forward, or a gruesome peril.

If a gene is inserted into cells growing in culture, there is potential for unlimited production of a particular *protein. The advantages in the case of insulin are obvious: human insulin is now available for treatment of diabetic patients, who cannot make their own. This product is particularly valuable for diabetics who are allergic to animal insulin. Pig insulin, which has been used for patients sensitive to the commonly used beef insulin, is being replaced by recombinant human insulin.

If a gene is inserted into the first cells of a newly conceived organism, some or all of the cells of that organism may make the product of the gene. In this way, a genetic defect could be rectified. It will take a long time to realize some of the possibilities. Certain inherited diseases of the blood are early targets for research, because it is technically possible to put genes into *stem cells taken from the *bone marrow, and return them to the host. In agriculture, new species of plants and animals can be made. Crops can be made resistant to disease. Extra copies of growth hormone genes have been inserted into fertilized pig ova, with the result that the pigs grow faster and bigger. Moreover, the offspring of these pigs inherit the faster growth.

For cancer, the first benefit of genetic engineering is the production of *growth factors. The while cell growth factors *G-CSF and *GM-CSF are being introduced to overcome the inhibition of white blood cell production caused by medications used in *chemotherapy. *Erythropoietin, a growth factor for red blood cells, offers relief of symptoms caused by *anaemia in cancer. Early studies of *interleukin-2, a growth factor produced by certain white cells, have shown regressions of cancer in a proportion of advanced cases. It is suggested, but not yet proved, that these regressions result from activation of immune cells that destroy cancer cells.

gene probing technique for demonstrating the presence of a *gene in *cells or *tissues.

genome the whole set of *genes possessed by an individual. Every person inherits his genes from his parents. The genes (sentences) are written in the *genetic code, strung together on *chromosomes (chapters). The genome constitutes the whole book or blueprint of life. Cancer results from falsification of the genome.

geographical distribution of cancer By finding places in the world where particular cancers are frequent and by studying local conditions, it has been possible to identify cancer-producing habits, lifestyles that favour development of cancer, and environmental carcinogens. There are astonishing differences in the incidence of particular cancers in different parts of the world. For example, the incidence of cancer of the *oesophagus in Iran is 300 times greater that in countries with the lowest incidence. Other ratios of highest to lowest incidence are: more than 200 for *skin cancer (highest rate in Australia), 100 for *liver cancer (parts of Africa) and 300 for penis (Uganda).

*Stomach cancer is responsible for 48% of all Japanese male cancer, compared to 7% of cancer in America and 4% in Australia. Stomach cancers are also common in the Soviet Union. The incidence of stomach cancer is declining almost everywhere, while the total incidence of cancer is increasing. Improvements in the preservation of food, particularly by refrigeration, are probably important in the decline of stomach cancer.

*Bowel cancer causes only half as many deaths in the Japanese as in Americans and other Western populations. The incidence of cancer of the large bowel is increasing in Japan and the Soviet Union. The incidence in the State of Connecticut is 10 times greater than in low risk countries in Africa. Bowel cancers were uncommon in Greek communities living in Australia, but have become more common the longer migrants have lived in Australia.

Women have a low incidence of *breast cancer in Japan, but women born in the USA of Japanese parents have the same high incidence of breast cancer as other women in the USA. Japanese men have a low incidence of *prostate cancer and a similar increase in prostatic carcinoma occurs in Japanese men born in USA.

All these geographical differences in the incidence of particular cancers point to *diet as a major factor responsible for the difference.

Of course, other factors may operate as well. Incidence of *breast cancer in Shanghai is one-fifth that in USA. Among Shanghai women, a long period of breast feeding (nine or more cumulative years) reduces the incidence even further, to only one third of that in Chinese women who have never breast-fed.

The oesophagus (the 'gullet') takes food from the mouth to the stomach. *Oesophageal cancer occurs frequently along the shores of the Caspian Sea and in some regions of China. Food moulds and a deficiency of *vitamin A are suspected factors.

Australia has the highest incidence of *malignant melanoma in the world, because it is the closest country to the equator having a large white-skinned population. Mediterranean immigrants have much lower rates and *skin cancers are almost unknown among Aborigines. Australia also has the highest incidence of *mesothelioma.

Gissmann, Lutz contemporary German virologist, Professor in Heidelberg, who developed the technique for demonstration of *human papilloma viruses (HPV) in cells of the human cervix

glioma   type of *brain cancer

Goiânia   city in Brazil, where dumped radioactive waste caused deaths. See *atomic bombs and nuclear reactors

grief   see *bereavement

growth   increase in number of *cells, resulting from cell division. Tissues grow if cell division exceeds cell death. See *nature of cancer.

growth factor   cell product that influences growth of tissue. Growth factors are typically broken down rapidly in the body, so that they only exert an influence at short range. *Hormones, on the other hand, are produced by glands in one part of the body and, by entering the circulation, may exert an influence on tissues throughout the body. See *nature of cancer.

White blood cell growth factors made in the laboratory by *genetic engineering are becoming available to help patients overcome the depression of white cell production caused by cancer *chemotherapy. They are effective if given in doses large enough to compensate for their short lives in the body. *G-CSF and *GM-CSF are the first of these to become available.

H

haemorrhoid   varicose veins of the lower end of the bowel, that may bleed. See *bowel cancer.

hairy cell leukaemia   rare *leukaemia caused by a virus (human T cell leukaemia virus II)

half-life   time for radioactive material to lose half of its radioactivity. For example, *iodine-131 emits only half as much *radiation after 8 days and only one quarter as much after 16 days. Each radioactive element has its own half-life, which never varies. The half-lives of radioactive elements range from seconds to years. Elements with long half-lives present the greatest danger from *atomic bombs and nuclear accidents.

Halotestin   trade name of *fluoxymesterone.

HEAD AND NECK CANCER
Cancers occur in the skin, mouth, pharynx (region at the back of the mouth), larynx (voicebox), the nasal air sinuses and the salivary glands. Most are squamous cell cancers, like the common *skin cancer type.

Cancers of the mouth and tongue spread locally and to the *lymph nodes of the neck, causing lumps. They also spread to distant parts, such as the lung, in some patients.

Causes of Head and Neck Cancer
Cancers of the mouth is relatively infrequent in people in Western societies who do not use *tobacco in any form, and who do not drink concentrated alcoholic spirits. For people smoking two packs of cigarettes per day, the risk of developing head and neck cancer is two to five times that of nonsmokers. *Alcohol, particularly spirits, increases the risk of head and neck cancer by 3 to 11 times. For persons who both smoke and drink alcohol, the risk is 15 to 16 times greater than for nonsmokers. This type of cancer is common in parts of the world where betel or tobacco is chewed, or snuff is taken. Poor oral and dental hygiene are probably factors in all populations.

*Nasopharyngeal carcinoma, occurring most commonly in Asia, is associated with infection by the *Epstein-Barr virus and *nitrosamines in salted fish. Other factors that predispose to head and neck cancer include *ultraviolet light from the sun, (*skin cancer, including lip cancer), *asbestos (*larynx cancer), work in the shoe, woodworking, textile and *nickel industries (cancer of the nasal cavity and nasal sinuses, see *occupation and cancer). Cancer of the mouth occurs with increased frequency in persons who have *coeliac disease and in persons chronically deficient in *iron. Head and neck cancers have been reported in young people who smoke *marijuana, but there is no proof marijuana causes cancer. A *diet high in fruits and vegetable and *vitamins A and *C appears to offer protection against development of cancer of the mouth.

Symptoms of Head and Neck Cancer
Cancers of the oral cavity appear as lumps, thickening, ulcers or sores that do not heal, in cheeks, gums, mouth and tongue. Early diagnosis is very important. Unfortunately a high proportion of these cancers are neglected or not treated, with the result that 80 per cent of patients with late cancers at the time of detection are dead within 18 months. Males are affected by oral cancer twice as often as females, mostly those over the age of 45. One third of people who seek advice about sores or lumps in the mouth that are malignant, go first to a dentist.

Thinning of the lining *epithelium in the mouth and abnormal whitish coloration, called *leukoplakia, may precede the development of cancer. Sometimes warty outgrowths are the first sign.

Treatment of Head and Neck Cancer
Treatment of cancers of the oral cavity demands a team approach for best results. *Surgery, *radiotherapy and *chemotherapy all have their place. In small tumours, surgery or radiotherapy may be curative. In other cases, chemotherapy may convert a cancer from being inoperable to being operable.

Chemotherapy is becoming more effective in these cases, and now some patients who were previously incurable are surviving. Radiotherapy is often used as well as chemotherapy.

help In Australia and most Western countries, *Anti-cancer Societies and Foundations are highly developed. These bodies exist to fight cancer by research, education and various patient services. Patients are urged to telephone or visit the foundation in their city to obtain information and solutions to various needs. Addresses and telephone numbers of Australian anti-cancer societies are listed in the Appendix.

The cancer services of University Teaching Hospitals have resources to help with may cancer-associated problems. For example, for patients who are not well enough to cope at the moment, or spouses who need respite, arrangements can be made for respite care. Doctors who are not actually members of the Hospital cancer service can arrange for consultations. See *coping with cancer.

hepatitis B virus (HBV) cause of hepatitis and a causal factor in *liver cancer. See *viruses and cancer.

hepatoma   alternative name for primary *liver cancer

heptachlor   *chlorinated insecticide

herbal teas   see *tea

heredity and cancer   Heredity appears to play a relatively small part in predisposing to the common cancers, but a dominant part in the incidence of some rare cancers. Some of these rare conditions have been very important in helping scientists to understand the processes which lead to the development of common cancers.

In *retinoblastoma, a malignant tumour develops at the back of the eye in children. The tendency to develop retinoblastoma is inherited. Both parents must have the *gene, although neither may develop the condition. The affected child inherits two faulty genes, one from each parent. Retinoblastoma also occurs sporadically, in subjects with no family history of the disease.

*Neurofibromatosis or von Recklinghausen's syndrome is a relatively common disorder, occurring in 1 in 3000 persons, characterized by pigmented skin patches together with little harmless tumours of nerves under the skin. There is a 50% risk that each offspring of an affected patient will have patches of pigmentation of skin tumours. Sometimes these tumours become malignant.

In *Down's syndrome, which used to be called mongolism, there is a 30–fold increase in the risk of *leukaemia. Down's syndrome is caused by an extra *chromosome in a faulty ovum.

In the rare *Bloom's syndrome and *xeroderma pigmentosum affected individuals die young from a variety of cancers. The importance of these rare conditions is that they have shown one way in which a hereditary defect can cause cancer. The defect is an inability to repair naturally occurring damage to the hereditary material *DNA. Subjects with these conditions usually die from *skin cancers, because *ultraviolet light in sunlight is very damaging to DNA. Those who avoid sunlight, but smoke, usually die in their 20s from *lung cancer. See *mutation.

In the condition *coeliac disease, there is a tendency to develop *lymphomas, cancers of the *mouth and *oesophagus. Coeliac disease is linked to the inheritance of certain blood groups from each parent. The condition is usually not evident in the parents.

Heredity may have a weak influence on the chance of developing some common cancers. The risk of *breast cancer is increased for women whose mother or sisters have had a breast cancer. The chance of cancer developing is also increased in persons having a family history cancer of the large *bowel, cancer of the lining of the *uterus (the endometrium) and *malignant melanoma. A tendency to develop melanomas is also associated with the *dysplastic naevus syndrome.

heroin   narcotic drug of the morphine family, once considered the most potent agent for control of pain, but according to the National Health and Medical Research Council of Australia, 'having no demonstrable advantage in the relief of chronic severe pain which cannot be obtained through other regimens of pain control widely available'.

Hiroshima   Japanese city destroyed by an atomic bomb in World War II, on 6 August 1945. See *atomic bombs and nuclear reactors.

Hodgkin, Thomas   1798–1866, English physician, who described a number of cases of enlargement of lymph nodes that had features distinct from diseases recognized at that time. Hodgkin worked at Guy's Hospital, London, where he was a lecturer in pathology and later practiced in St Thomas's Hospital. See *Hodgkin's disease.

Hodgkin's disease   the most frequent form of *lymphoma occurring in Western society, named after Thomas *Hodgkin. Once considered incurable, Hodgkin's disease represents a triumph of modern medicine, because not only can it be be cured at an early stage by *radiotherapy, but also patients with relatively advanced disease may be cured by *chemotherapy. See *lymphoma.

hormone   gland product that controls growth and function of other tissues. Hormones reach target tissues via the circulation. Hormones are used to control *breast cancer, *prostate cancer, *lymphoma and *leukaemia.

hormone replacement therapy   treatment with *oestrogen, or oestrogen plus *progestin, after the menopause, for life.
   The average woman in the Western world is postmenopausal for one third of her life. After the menopause, the bones of women become thinner and they undergo other changes associated with ageing. Loss of bone mass leads to the relatively high risk of fractures in later life. The only way this can be stopped is by taking sex hormones, and in the case of women this effectively means oestrogens, although exercise definitely slows the loss of bone strength.
   After the menopause oestrogens also have a preventative effect on blood vessel disease, because they reverse the change in hormonal balance towards the male, low oestrogen condition that favours *arteriosclerosis. Therefore, many obstetricians are advising women to take oestrogenic medications for the rest of their lives after the menopause.
   One study claims that the long-term use of oestrogens by postmenopausal women adds four years to a woman's life expectancy, mainly through reduction of heart disease. There are no studies on the benefits of taking progestins as well. Results of 20 different

studies did not show that oestrogen was associated with breast cancer, indicating that the risks are not great. However, in a very large study, involving 23,244 Swedish women, published in August 1989, oestradiol, a particular type of oestrogen, nearly doubled the risk of breast cancer after 9 years of use.

This study illustrates some of the difficulties of getting at the essential truth, sorting out the wheat from the chaff. Because the investigators did not know how many years these women had been taking contraceptive oestrogen preparations before the menopause, we do not know if the risk was related to previous use of the pill. Some of the women may have previously taken the earlier high-dose type of contraceptives for many years. The same uncertainty exists with regard to the risk of *uterus (endometrium) cancer.

The benefit from the use of oestrogens after the menopause must be balanced against the side effects of the treatment. It has been estimated that for every woman who might lose her life from breast cancer because of long-term use of oestrogen, another seven might be spared premature death from heart attack or stroke. It is quite unclear at present whether the other type of female hormone, *progestin, counteracts or enhances the cancer-producing effects of oestrogen. Studies are in progress, but these cannot help women until they have been published.

The best opinion today is that these benefits of oestrogen outweigh the cancer risks, but no unqualified guarantee of the safety of hormonal replacement therapy can be given at present. Recently the Lancet has stated that the addition of a progestin '(given for a minimum of 12 days each month) to the continuous oestrogen treatment is mandatory in women who have not had a hysterectomy, to prevent endometrial hyperplasia. This treatment usually results in a regular withdrawal bleed which becomes less well tolerated with increasing age. . . Moreover, since the very long-term safety of hormone replacement has not yet been fully elucidated, there is a need for other effective therapies for the treatment of osteoporosis.'

hospice   very old term applying once to a house of rest for travellers, now used to designate a place for persons in advanced illness, particularly cancer. As well as offering accommodation, care and comfort, hospices organize home care and domestic help for families and patients.

*Anti-cancer Societies can help with addresses of hospices.

human immunodeficiency virus (HIV)   *virus causing *AIDS.

human papilloma virus (HPV)   very large family of *viruses causing *warts, including genital warts. Causative factor of *cervix cancer.

human T Cell leukaemia virus I (HTLV-1)   *virus causing *adult T cell leukaemia (ATL).

hyperthermia   Cancer cells appear unable to resist high temperatures. Normal cells can remain alive at 41°C, whereas cancer cells die.

Although it sounds a simple treatment, it is in fact difficult to raise the temperature of cancer cells without generally raising the temperature of the body, or of a large volume of tissue around the cancer. Of course the temperature of the whole body cannot be raised to 41°C.

An ingenious way is being developed to treat brain tumours by hyperthermia. Magnetic metal seeds inserted into the brain can be moved into place by external magnets. When the seeds are placed strategically in the tumour, the heat can be applied by appropriate radiation that is picked up by the seeds. *Lasers can also be used to induce local hyperthermia.

Hyperthermia has been used in conjunction with *radiotherapy with variable results.

Hydrea   trade name of hydroxyurea, medication used in cancer *chemotherapy

hydroxyurea   medication used in cancer *chemotherapy

hysterectomy   surgical removal of the uterus

Ichikawa, Kiyoshi born 1878, Japanese eye specialist, who studied in Germany and became professor in Kyoto. With *Yamagiwa, he showed that *tar painted on the skin of rabbits caused cancers.

immune system widerspread system of cells found in *lymphoid tissues, capable of seeking out and destroying foreign cells or their products. The immune system forms the defence force of the body against disease-causing microorganisms.

immunity and cancer The immune system protects us from invasion by foreign organisms — viruses, bacteria, fungi, free living single-cell animals like amoebae and even parasitic worms. The system consists of widespread *lymphoid tissues containing a variety of specialized cells. The immune defence force has two arms, *antibodies and specialized *cells. Antibodies are *proteins with a shape that precisely fits part of the target. By binding to a microorganism, antibodies can disarm it, so that a cell of the immune system can destroy it. Antibodies can deal with poisons from foreign organisms in the same way. Other specialized cells of the immune system can directly attack the invading organisms without help from antibodies.

It has been asked for a long time whether the immune system can protect us from cancers, enemy cells from within. There is no longer any doubt that it can, but if a cancer gets beyond a minimum size, the immune defence mechanisms can no longer cope. Persons whose immune defences are impaired, for example as a result of particular diseases, including *AIDS, are prone to develop *skin cancers, *lymphomas and other cancers.

Much research effort is being expended to devise strategies that will overcome the resistance of larger tumours to the body's defences. Immune cells of the *lymphocyte class can be harvested from the blood or from a tumour for culture in the laboratory, away from the unfavourable conditions of the battle zone. They will multiply under suitable conditions, in the presence of the *growth factor *interleukin-2, until they number billions. When they are returned to the patient, they are able to kill off a very large proportion of the cancer cells.

This type of treatment is yet to cure, but does seem to produce very big reductions in particular tumours, particularly *malignant melanomas and *kidney cancers.

Use of antibodies to fight cancer is in its early stages. A single cell which produces the required antibody can be fused with an immortal cancer cell in the test tube. This hybrid cell becomes the parent of unlimited numbers of antibody-producing cells (hence the term *'monoclonal antibody'). In some instances it is possible to produce antibodies which combine with a structure on a cancer cell. Such cancer-specific antibodies can be linked to an anticancer drug. When the antibody-drug complex is injected into the patient, the antibody becomes a deadly messenger, delivering the drug directly to the cancer cells. Alternatively, the antibody can be made radioactive, so that it can deliver a fatal dose of X-rays to tumour cells. Radioactive antibodies can also be used to detect hidden deposits of cancer cells. At present most successful systems produce mouse antibodies, which are therefore foreign to humans and may cause allergic reactions.

Radioactive monoclonal antibodies have been used to purge bone marrow of cancer cells for *bone marrow transplantation in patients with *Hodgkin's disease and *lymphoma. Blood-forming cells are first aspirated from the bone marrow and treated with radioactive monoclonal antibody. After the patient has been treated with high doses of *chemotherapy, the purged bone marrow, now free of cancer cells, is returned to the patient.

Sometimes the pathologist can diagnose cancer under the microscope, but he cannot tell the type. Monoclonal antibodies against different types of cell, labelled with a stain, have proved very valuable for classifying cancers.

A patient whose *immune system is not functioning well because of the effects of *chemotherapy, or because the disease involves the immune system itself, can often be given very effective protection from common infections by regular injections of *gamma globulin, a preparation containing anti-microbial antibodies from the blood of normal subjects.

immunotherapy   treatment designed to control cancer by enhancing the capacity of natural immune defence mechanisms to destroy cancer cells, just as they destroy infectious microorganisms.

Some *alternative cancer treatments are called immunotherapy, without much evidence that they influence the immune system.

impotence   inability to perform the sexual act, a problem in debilitated states and sometimes a problem in particular cancers. The term refers particularly to inability of men to obtain or maintain an erection, but loss of desire also affects women. Other aspects of the sexual act are often affected, including loss of lubrication function in women, inability to achieve orgasm, premature ejaculation and absence of emission.

*Androgen deficiency in treated patients with *prostate cancer causes loss of desire and failure of emission associated with lack of seminal fluid. Premature ejaculation and absence of orgasm are usually due to anxiety or a state of depression. Other psychological factors cause impotence, such as worry, fatigue, marital discord or lack of interest in the partner. Also many drugs cause impotence, including

Incidence of cancer

sedatives, tranquillisers, alcohol and narcotics. Sometimes the blood supply to the penis is reduced by *arteriosclerosis.

Specialist help may be needed to diagnose the cause of impotence. By far the commonest causes are psychological factors, ill health and drugs. Treatment depends on the cause. As an example, a women with breast cancer reported to her doctor that she had trouble with her marriage and wondered if she had become frigid or her husband impotent. Sexual relations with her husband had stopped after mastectomy. Careful examination of the circumstances and an interview with her husband revealed that he had had irrational anger and feelings of worthlessness when his wife's illness became known. The marriage had been unusually close and he could not bear the thought of her death. Through discussion, explanation that many spouses of patients with serious diseases have similar feelings, and judicious counselling, the husband was able to overcome his feelings, the situation was resolved and he could be helpful to her through her terminal illness. See *testis, *prostate cancer.

incidence of cancer the occurrence of cancer, usually expressed as a proportion of the population. The incidence of different types (Table 8) differs greatly from the *mortality as shown in Table 10. The relative incidence of cancers is discussed under *sites of cancer. See also Table 9 in *magnitude of the cancer problem.

Table 8: Incidence of different types of cancer

Number of persons in each 100,000 of the population who contract particular cancers each year

Type	Males	Females
Breast		79
Lung	65	21
Large Bowel	59	53
Prostate	66	
Melanoma	26	29
Stomach	15	8
Lymphoma	18	15
Leukaemia	16	10
Cervix		15
Uterus (Endometrium)		16
Ovary		10
Pancreas	10	8
Kidney and ureters	12	7
Brain	8	5
Multiple Myeloma	3	3
All Sites	395	334

These 1987 figures are from the South Australian Cancer Registry and are representative of Western societies.

infertility   see *chemotherapy: fertility, infertility and pregnancy in; *testis cancer

injury in causation of cancer   Patients frequently attribute the development of a cancer to an injury. A patient with a bone tumour is likely to remember a blow of some sort to the involved part. A blow to the head has frequently been blamed for the onset of a brain tumour.

If injury to any part of the body were shown to play a causative role in cancer, the implications would be enormous. Employers would have to shoulder a huge liability for compensation, and lifestyles would have to be changed to avoid injury.

Fortunately, there is no good evidence supporting a relationship between simple physical injury and cancer. Sports injuries have not led to such a suspicion and no increase of cancer has been reported during war time, or from war injuries.

On the other hand certain kinds of repeated injury may cause cancer. Skin cancer in Kashmir is caused by hot earthenware warming pots. Malignant change sometimes occurs in chronic ulcers of the lower leg. Occasionally skin cancers occur in burn scars.

interferon   class of *growth factors discovered during investigation of defences against viral infections. Besides their protective action against viruses, interferons regulate growth under some circumstances. Interferon made by *gene technology is used to treat several types of cancer, particularly chronic myeloid *leukaemia, in which cures have been reported. Responses are also obtained in another rare type of leukaemia (*hairy cell leukaemia), in some *lymphomas and in *malignant melanoma.

interleukin-2   white cell *growth factor used to produce large numbers of tumour-fighting immune cells. The immune cells are taken from the patient's tumour, cultured in the laboratory in the presence of nutrients and interleukin-2, then returned to the patient by a vein. Also used in cancer therapy by injection into patients, on an experimental basis.

iron deficiency   of a chronic nature predisposes to cancer of the oesophagus. Persons may become deficient in iron because their diet is inadequate, through bowel disease resulting in poor absorption, or through loss of blood. Iron is needed by all *cells, particularly red blood cells.

isotretinoin   *retinoid-type medication

J

jaundice yellow discolouration of skin and eyes due to accumulation of bile pigments normally excreted by the liver. Jaundice can be caused by liver disease, by obstruction of the bile duct or by excessive breakdown of red blood cells, from which bile pigments are made.

Jenner, Sir Edward 1749–1823, Gloucestershire doctor who induced infection with cowpox for immunisation against smallpox, demonstrating protective power of *vaccines. In 1796 he took pus from the sore of a dairy maid and inoculated James Phipps, a healthy boy of eight. The boy developed a small pustule. Six weeks later Jenner inoculated him with smallpox exudate and he did not develop smallpox. After repeating the experiment successfully on three more subjects he published his work. Such a small series aroused much controversy, but various famous people soon had the vaccination and Jenner himself became famous. The English Parliament voted him a total of 30,000 pounds, a fortune in those days.

K

Kaposi, Moritz 1837–1902, Viennese dermatologist, whose name is associated with *Kaposi's sarcoma

Kaposi's sarcoma formerly rare *skin cancer now occurring in patients with *AIDS

KIDNEY CANCER

Kidneys make urine by filtering out fluid from the blood, extracting from the fluid precious commodities for return to the blood and concentrating the urine to conserve the body's water. The fluid flows through tubes called ureters into the bladder.

Cause of Kidney Cancer
*Tobacco smoke, *aniline dye products, *aspirin and *phenacetin are thought to be factors in causing kidney tumours.

Symptoms of Kidney Cancer
The cardinal sign of cancer of the kidneys is passing blood in the urine. The finding of blood in the urine, even in minute quantities, is always a serious matter that must be investigated.

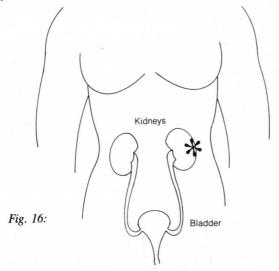

Fig. 16:

Kidneys

Bladder

Cancer of the kidney. Urine formed in the kidneys flows through the ureters into the bladder. Cancer of the kidney often comes to notice by blood in the urine.

Kidney cancer

Blood often does not enter the urine until the cancer is large. When it does, the patient may become tired because of *anaemia. Sometimes the cancer makes chemical substances that cause fever. The first symptoms may result from seedlings in the lungs or elsewhere.

Diagnosis of Kidney Cancer

Blood can enter the urine from anywhere in the urinary tract—from the kidneys, ureters, bladder or from the urethra, the tube leading from the bladder to the outside of the body. The source of blood in the urine is found by *pyelograms, *X-rays, *ultrasound examination and *endoscopy.

Treatment of Kidney Cancer

Removal of the affected kidney will cure the patient if the cancer has not spread. Widespread cancer of the kidney often does not respond to any treatment. Remarkable cures are seen from time to time from the use of the *progestin type hormones. Some patients experience a response to the new agent *interferon.

*Wilms' tumour is a cancer of the kidney that occurs in children. Though this was previously considered an incurable cancer, 75% of patients are now cured by combination of *surgery, *radiotherapy and *chemotherapy.

L

laetrile also known as amygdalin and krebiozen, chemical substance widely claimed to benefit cancer patients, now shown by exhaustive public enquiries to be without effect as a cancer treatment. Under some circumstances laetrile is quite toxic. See *alternative cancer treatments.

laparoscope *endoscope inserted through the abdominal wall for examining the contents of the abdomen

laparotomy operation to open the abdomen

LARYNX CANCER
Cancer of the larynx, or voice box, mainly affects the vocal cords.

Cause of Cancer of the Larynx
This cancer occurs mainly in *tobacco smokers.

Symptoms of Cancer of the Larynx
Larynx cancer causes hoarseness, a symptom which must therefore not be neglected.

Diagnosis of Cancer of the Larynx
The larynx can be inspected by specialists with the aid of a mirror, without the need for general anaesthesia.

Treatment of Cancer of the Larynx
Treatment depends on the size and spread of the cancer. If found early, it may be cured by *surgery and *radiotherapy can cure cases that are not too advanced. Larynx cancer spreads locally, to *lymph nodes in the neck and by the blood to distant parts of the body. *Chemotherapy may benefit patients whose disease is inoperable.

laser instrument to produce an intense beam of pure light. Laser is an acronym for light amplification by stimulated emission of *radiation. Different types produce light of different wavelengths, including ultraviolet and infrared light.
Many kinds of lasers offer advantages or potential benefit in the treatment of cancer. Carbon dioxide lasers can be used as sophisticated scalpels to cut tissue, at the same time sealing bleeding points. They are valuable for treatment of cancer of the *cervix, cancer of the *mouth and in other sites.
Nd-YAG (Neodymium, yttrium aluminium garnet) lasers produce great heat and can obliterate cancers that are obstructing the large

airways of the *lung. This treatment brings great relief from distressing symptoms, but does not cure the cancers. The YAG laser appears to be especially useful for treatment of tumours in infants because it can prevent excessive blood loss and can excise tumours cleanly when they are close to small organs and vessels that might be damaged by other surgical techniques.

The output from an Nd-Yag laser can be funnelled via a light-transmitting fibre into the centre of tumours. If the laser light is applied at low power, there is gentle heating resulting in killing by *hyperthermia. As long as the heat applied is not excessive, the surrounding normal tissue is undamaged. The dead tumour can be left where it is and the body's healing mechanisms will remove the debris and replace it either with scar tissue or regenerated normal tissue. This technique is in the experimental stage for the treatment of humans with *liver tumours.

Lasers can be used to treat cancer by a technique known as *photo-dynamic therapy. In this treatment the patient is first injected with a light-sensitive substance that becomes concentrated in most types of cancer. Two or three days later, laser light of the appropriate wavelength is directed to the tumour. The light activates the light-sensitive substance in the tumour to release toxic oxygen molecules that kill cancer cells.

Photodynamic therapy is still in the developmental stages. It can be used to treat early lung cancers when the patient is not able to undergo an operation involving the removal of one or more segments of lung tissue. It shows promise in the treatment of *brain tumours, when used together with surgery and radiotherapy. It is effective in treatment of *skin cancers.

LEUKAEMIA

Leukaemias are cancers of white cells that circulate in the blood, often in vast numbers. There are many types of leukaemia, which vary greatly from one another in the symptoms they cause, their curability and the course of the disease.

There are also considerable differences between the leukaemias of children and those affecting adults. Approximately one child in 3000 develops leukaemia before his or her tenth birthday. **Acute lymphoblastic leukaemia** is the commonest childhood malignancy.

The major division in the leukaemias is into the acute and the chronic types. Acute leukaemias occur predominantly in children and young adults, developing rapidly and progressing fatally unless treated. Immature cells are seen in the blood, often in low numbers. The chronic leukaemias occur mainly in adults and are of two major types, myeloid, of white blood cells born in the *bone marrow, and lymphoid, of white cells born in the *lymphoid tissues. High numbers of relatively mature white cells circulate in the blood. The chronic types are virtually never curable. In children, the cure rate in acute leukaemia ranges from over 50% to 75%, depending on the type. In adults the cure rates are not so high: even in the adult leukaemias with the most favourable prognosis, treated in the best centres, less than 40% are free of leukaemia after 5 years.

The bone marrow is always invaded by leukaemic cells, which crowd the normal blood-forming cells and impair the production of normal red cells, causing *anaemia, and of white cells, resulting in susceptibility to infections, and *platelets, leading to a bleeding tendency.

Cause of Leukaemias

Some leukaemias are caused by *radiations, *benzene and anti-cancer drugs (see *medical treatment as a cause of cancer). Persons with *Down's syndrome are predisposed to leukaemia. Human T cell Leukaemia Virus I (HTLV-I) causes leukaemias and *lymphomas in Japan, the Caribbean and Africa, as well as sporadic cases in Western countries.

Symptoms of Leukaemia

Patients experience loss of energy, sometimes bleeding and are often prone to infections. A blood test shows numerous abnormal white cells and the *diagnosis is confirmed by examining cells of the bone marrow.

Treatment of Leukaemia

Because leukaemic cells travel in the blood leukaemia cannot be treated by surgery or radiotherapy. Until *chemotherapy was developed, there was little to offer. Now remissions can be obtained in more than 90% of children with **acute lymphoblastic leukaemia.** Cure is now achieved in over 50% of all types of childhood leukaemia. The key to curing childhood acute lymphoblastic leukaemia is adequate initial treatment, which must be carried out in a centre that specializes in treatment of the condition.

The chronic leukaemias of adults can often be controlled very well for many years. **Chronic lymphocytic leukaemia** is usually a disease of older persons and it is often so slowly progressive that it does not affect the lifespan of the patient. In fact, treatment is often quite unnecessary and possibly detrimental in many patients with this type of leukaemia. Treatment is required if symptoms are troublesome or if the disease begins to advance rapidly.

It is now common practice to take bone marrow, early in the course of the disease, for storage at very low temperatures. Deep frozen marrow can be stored for at least ten years and returned when the remaining bone marrow is no longer meeting the patient's needs, usually because of the effect of chemotherapy.

Leukoplakia

*Bone marrow transplantation is being used increasingly in the treatment of leukaemia, to enable high doses of cancer chemotherapeutic agents, which severely damage the bone marrow, to be given.

Patients with leukaemia, particularly chronic lymphocytic leukaemia and those whose immune defences are weakened by chemotherapy, can be protected from common infections by injections of *gamma globulin.

A rare kind of leukaemia of the lymphoid type, called **hairy cell leukaemia** has become a landmark condition, because it is dramatically controlled by a new drug, *interferon.

leukoplakia   whitish thickening of mouth or other mucous membrane that can be a precancerous or the site of actual cancer. Leukoplakia should always be investigated by *biopsy.

Lifestyle and Cancer

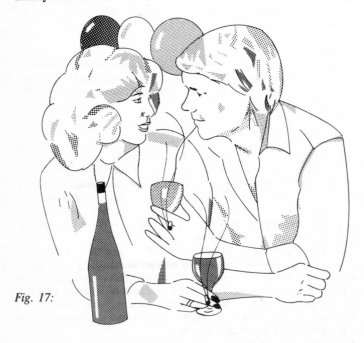

Fig. 17:

Lifestyle and cancer. Our chances of developing cancer are largely determined by the way we live. Lifestyle includes diet, occupation, recreational drugs and the environment in which we live.

Lifestyle may be defined as all of the factors involved in the way people live, including their habits, where they live, their work, the *air they breathe, the *water they drink and what they put in it. *Diet is a major factor in lifestyle. It is hard to conceive of all the activities that are encompassed by the term 'lifestyle', particularly when we try to analyse which of the lifestyle factors may cause a particular cancer. It is also hard to realize how much life has changed in the past 75 years. This period has seen the introduction of electricity supplies, automobiles, refrigeration, antibiotics, modern surgery, hundreds of thousands of new chemical substances and complex changes to the environment.

It is these changes in lifestyle, resulting from the applications of scientific discoveries and from the changes in social outlook, that have resulted in remarkable prolongation of human life. However, it is generally believed by the leading epidemiologists that lifestyle factors account for more than three quarters of cancers. Cancer mortality attributed to tobacco amounts to about 30%, to diet 35%, to reproductive and sexual factors 8% and to occupational factors 4%.

Now that we know that most cancers are avoidable, we must analyse lifestyles for the factors that cause cancer. *Socioeconomic class strongly influences lifestyle and the incidence of some cancers, such as *stomach and *cervix cancers, has been related to socioeconomic class.

lindane   *chlorinated insecticide

LIVER CANCER
In Western countries, most cancers that involve the liver are *metastases from cancers that start in other organs. Cancers of *bowel, *breast, *lung, *pancreas and *lymphomas are prone to spread to the liver.

Cause of Liver Cancer
Globally speaking, most primary cancers of the liver (hepatomas) are caused by the *hepatitis B virus. About 20% of the Chinese population are chronically infected with the hepatitis B virus, compared to less than 1% of the population of developed countries. In Taiwan the major cancer is cancer of the liver. A large *epidemiological study in Taiwan by the American R Palmer *Beasley showed that cancer of the liver occurred almost exclusively in carriers of the hepatitis B virus and the same is believed to be true for mainland China.

A second major factor in the development of liver cancer, particularly in Africa, is *aflatoxin, a contaminant of mouldy peanuts. Aflatoxin and hepatitis B virus frequently act together in inducing hepatoma.

115

Liver cancer

The other major cause of liver cancer is *alcohol. In Western countries, primary liver cancer is a disease of chronic alcoholics. A rare cause, now presumably eliminated by rigorous control of exposure to it, is *vinyl chloride monomer, a hazard to workers in the manufacture of plastics, which led to a rare type of liver cancer. See *chemicals as causes of cancer.

Symptoms of Liver Cancer
Cancers in the liver may cause no symptoms until they have reached considerable size. As the liver supplies energy in the form of sugar and fat, involvement of the liver by cancer usually results in loss of energy and tiredness. Pain is uncommon. *Jaundice occurs late in the condition because the liver can no longer excrete the coloured waste products from old red blood cells.

Treatment of Liver Cancer
Large tumours of the liver or multiple metastases of most cancers are incurable. Advances have been made in surgical removal of liver tumours, particularly since *computed tomography has permitted accurate assessment and localization of tumours in the liver. Deposits of *lymphoma and some cancers respond to *chemotherapy.

Prevention of Liver Cancer
Both infection with hepatitis B virus and resulting liver cancer may be prevented by effective hepatitis virus B *vaccination. It has been shown in China that without immunization 10% of babies are already chronically infected by the first year of life. Ninety per cent of infants born to mothers who carry the virus become infected. In trial vaccination programmes the number of chronically infected babies has been reduced to 1%.

According to Dr Beasley, there are no exceptions, throughout the entire world, to the relationship between high incidence of hepatitis B infection and a high incidence of primary cancer of the liver. Immunization could reduce total mortality in China and Taiwan by 20%. Like smallpox, which has been eradicated, hepatitis B is an eradicable disease.

In Western countries, in which hepatitis B is not endemic, liver cancer can be prevented by control of alcohol intake.

lomustine   medication used in cancer *chemotherapy

loss of hair   see *chemotherapy, side effects of

lumpectomy   operation to remove *breast cancer and surrounding tissue, without removing the whole breast

LUNG CANCER

Tumours of the lung are often *metastases from cancers originating in other organs. Primary cancers of the lung arise in the *epithelium of the airways of the lung.

Primary lung cancer is the commonest cause of cancer death in men and the second commonest in women. Now that men are smoking less and women are smoking more, there is a small fall in lung cancer deaths in older men, but lung cancer deaths are increasing in women by 5% each year. The incidence of lung cancer in non-smokers has risen 15–30–fold this century, particularly in people over 65 years of age.

There are three main types of lung cancer: **squamous cell cancer, adenocarcinoma** and **small cell carcinoma.** They all arise in the *epithelium lining the bronchi, the air tubes of the lung. Adenocarcinoma is the predominant cancer in non-smokers. Small cell carcinoma is incurable, no matter how small the tumour when it is detected, because the cancer spreads to other tissues very early.

If diagnosed early enough, adenocarcinoma and squamous cell carcinoma may be cured by surgical removal of the bronchus and the part of the lung it serves. About 10% of all patients survive 5 years. The others die, mostly in the first one to two years.

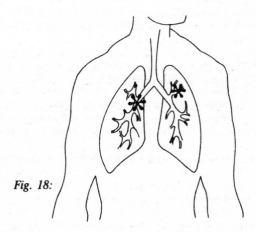

Fig. 18:

Lung cancers. Primary cancers of the lung arise from the airways. Sites of two cancers are illustrated (*), the larger arising from a main branch of the trachea (windpipe), another arising from a secondary branch.

Lung cancer

Causes of Lung Cancer
*Tobacco smoking is the principal cause of about 85% of lung cancers. *Passive smoking is held to be the cause of 17% of the lung cancers in non-smokers. Co-factors are involved in many cases. *Radon gas in houses is an important factor in some environments, also in mines, although it acts as co-factor with smoking in most cases. There is a significant risk of lung cancer in the *uranium industry. *Bischloromethyl ether, *asbestos, *chromium and *arsenic also cause lung cancer. *Air pollution from motor vehicle and industrial exhausts in cities is a small factor in the causation of lung cancer. See *occupation and cancer, *chemicals as causes of cancer.

Symptoms of Lung Cancer
The two cardinal symptoms of lung cancer are cough and coughing up of blood or blood-stained sputum. Smokers usually have a cough, although they are frequently unaware of it. Their spouses usually are! For this reason, smokers who have developed a cancer often come late for diagnosis. Sometimes the first hint of lung cancer is pneumonia in the part of the lung beyond the tumour. *Pain occurs when the lining of the lung (the *pleura) is involved.

Secondary cancers often cause no immediate problem and go unnoticed. As they enlarge they may cause shortness of breath and cough, particularly in patients with other lung diseases.

Chronic cough should always be investigated. Coughing of blood is more dramatic, usually leading the patients to seek medical advice without delay.

Diagnosis of Lung Cancer
Early cancers can only be demonstrated by *bronchoscopy, although cancer cells can be found in sputum by *cytology (that is, by special microscopic techniques). Later tumours may often be detected by X-ray of the chest. In Japan, mass surveys are conducted by people returning specimens of sputum to the laboratory in special containers.

The definitive diagnosis is made by microscopic examination of *biopsy specimens.

Treatment of Lung Cancer
Fewer than half of the patients with a lung cancer can be considered for *surgery with the intention of curing the disease. Of patients with potentially curable disease who continue to smoke, one third develop a second cancer.

Wherever possible, the patient is offered a chance of cure by *surgery, which is only possible if the tumour can be separated from vital organs within the chest. It entails removal of a segment or a lobe of a lung. The success rate is not high, for all types of lung cancer tend to spread early. Many patients have lungs so severely damaged

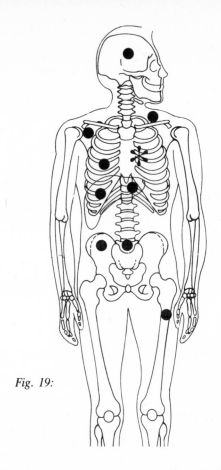

Fig. 19:

Spread of lung cancer. Seedlings from the primary tumour (*) may become tumours (●) in the liver, bones, brain, other parts of the lung and in the skin.

by many years of smoking that they could not survive the loss of lung tissue necessitated by the operation.

Small cell cancer of the lung usually responds very well to *chemotherapy. Unfortunately the control by chemotherapy rarely lasts more than a year. The other two types of lung cancer, which are the more common, usually do not respond adequately to the chemotherapy available at present.

It is rarely possible to offer patients the chance of surgical removal of secondary deposits, because the cancer has usually spread widely.

*Radiotherapy is used extensively for palliation of lung cancer. It controls pain from deposits in bones and pressure complications within the chest. Radiotherapy may also cure some early lung cancers of patients who are not fit for operation. *Laser treatment can play a valuable part in controlling distressing symptoms in patients who cannot be cured of lung cancer. Airways blocked by tumour can be cleared and bleeding can be stopped.

Prevention of Lung Cancer

By far the major measure to avoid lung cancer is to avoid smoking. Those who stop smoking immediately improve their risks and the reduction of risk continues steadily. After not smoking for ten years, those who had smoked 20 or less cigarettes a day have the same risk as nonsmokers of the same age. It takes 15 years for former heavier smokers to get back to the non-smoker's risk.

Workers in industries in which their *occupation entails a risk of lung cancer, particularly in the *uranium and *asbestos industries should on no account smoke, since they are at particularly high risk of developing lung cancer.

Recent evidence suggests that people who wish to give up smoking to improve their chances of avoiding cancer should also attend to their *diet. Many smokers appear to be low in vitamin A. This deficiency should be remedied by eating good food, containing *carotene, from which the body makes *vitamin A.

lymphocyte   class of wandering white blood cell that can make *antibodies. A member of the *immune system.

lymphoid tissues   large volume of tissues dispersed throughout the body, housing cells of the body's *immune system. Lymph nodes in the neck, abdomen, armpits and groins, as well as the spleen and tonsils, belong to this system. Lymph nodes are aggregates of cells of this system, ranging from pea to walnut size. Many of the white blood cells are made in these tissues. Lymph nodes filter the tissue fluid that is returning into the blood via *lymph vessels. Large aggregates of lymphoid tissue are in the wall of the bowel and in the airways of the lungs.

Many of the cells of this system roam the body in blood, lymph vessels and tissues, in search of foreign invaders. These foreign substances are usually microorganisms, but cells of the immune system also attack grafts of kidneys and other tissues.

LYMPHOMA

Lymphomas are malignant tumours of the cells of the *lymphoid tissues. There are many subtypes of lymphoma, corresponding to the many types of cell in lymphoid tissue.

Lymphomas have in common the propensity to spread to other *lymphoid tissue, to the *bone marrow and to the liver. In advanced cases the malignant tissue spreads very widely. Some types of lymphoma show important differences, particularly in response to treatment. In some rather rare types the skin is involved very early.

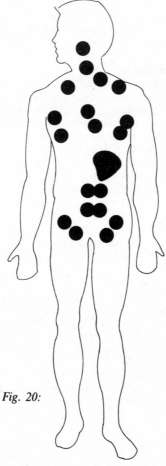

Fig. 20:

Lymph nodes are found in the neck, in the armpits, inside the chest at the roots of the lungs, in the abdomen alongside the backbone and adjacent to the bowel and in the groins. The tonsils are at the back of the mouth and the spleen is a larger organ in the left upper abdomen. Not shown are large amounts of lymphoid tissue in the wall of the bowel and the airways of the lungs.

Lymphoma

Cause of Lymphoma

The cause of lymphomas is not generally known. However, *Burkitt's lymphoma in tropical Africa is always associated with the *Epstein-Barr virus and lymphomas are sometimes caused by *chemotherapy and *X-rays. Lymphomas also arise in greater frequency in patients with *AIDS than in the general population and in patients whose immune system is defective for any reason, including those treated with drugs to control rejection of organ grafts (eg kidney, heart, liver). See *medical treatment as a cause of cancer.

Symptoms of Lymphoma

A lymphoma usually comes to notice as a painless lump in one or more lymph nodes. If the tumour arises in the abdomen it may not be found until it causes symptoms by pressure on abdominal structures.

Any lump that does not go down within a few days should be shown to the doctor. Lumps are not infrequent in lymph nodes of the neck as a result of a reaction to an infection, usually in the throat or tonsils. If such lumps do not go down within a week or two of treatment of infection, they must be examined by *biopsy.

When lymphoma involves the *bone marrow the patient has symptoms resulting from deficiency of the red and white cells and *platelets that are made there. Deficiency of red cells constitutes *anaemia. Deficiency of white cells leads to susceptibility to infections. The function of platelets is to prevent blood leaking from the small blood vessels, so patients lacking platelets tend to bleed.

Treatment of Lymphoma

The diagnosis of *Hodgkin's disease was considered a sentence of death three decades ago. The disease is of great historical importance, because Vera *Peters in Toronto showed in the 1950s that adequate doses of *radiotherapy were curative in a high proportion of cases. This was the first demonstration that cancers of the lymphoma class could be cured.

In the 1960s investigators in the National Cancer Institute, in the USA, introduced successful *chemotherapy for Hodgkin's disease, using four drugs in combination. This completely changed the outlook for patients who were not cured by radiotherapy and was the stimulus for the use of chemotherapy in other kinds of cancer.

Some of the lymphomas grow so slowly that it is often not necessary to treat them actively for a long time. Paradoxically, some of these slow-growing lymphomas are difficult to cure. By contrast, some of the fastest-growing lymphomas can actually be cured by chemotherapy alone. Lymphomas generally respond well to both chemotherapy and radiotherapy. The chance of complete remission, that is, destruction of all detectable tumour with a good probability of cure, even in advanced lymphoma, ranges between 40% and 80%.

Lymphomas are usually not cured by simple excision, because malignant cells wander very early in the course of the disease.

lymph nodes   see *lymphoid tissues

lymph stream   pathway of fluid from the tissues via lymphatic vessels, back to the blood. Lymph is filtered along the way in lymphoid tissues.

M

macrobiotic diet   see *alternative cancer treatments

magenta   a red dyestuff consisting of a mixture of *aniline dyes, also known as basic fuchsine. Magenta is used widely for staining tissue samples and bacteria. Magenta may cause cancer of the *bladder. See *occupation and cancer.

maglev trains   trains which are lifted from the rails by magnetic repulsion. See *power lines.

magnetic resonance imaging (MRI)   method of displaying pictures of body organs, based on detecting magnetic properties of atoms in the tissues

MAGNITUDE OF THE CANCER PROBLEM
There is no denying that the cancer problem is big. In 1987 when the world population was 5 billion there were about 5.9 million new cases of cancer in the world each year.

Cancer is now directly responsible each year for one fifth to one quarter of all deaths in Western countries. Cancer ranks second to heart disease, which causes about 38% of deaths. The other major causes of death are strokes (9%), accidents (5–6%), and lung disease and pneumonia (5%, at least half of which are related to tobacco).

Table 9: Numbers of cancers occurring worldwide in 1975

Type of cancer	Number (thousands)
Stomach	682
Lung	591
Breast	541
Colon/rectum	507
Cervix	459
Mouth/pharynx	340
Oesophagus	296
Liver	259
Lymphatic	221
Prostate	198
Bladder	176
Leukaemia	170
Other sites, by subtraction	1430
All sites, other than skin	5870

As estimated by Parkin, Sternswärd and Muir (1984)

About 900,000 new cases of cancer are diagnosed in the USA annually, amounting to about 3,500 cases per million. These figures do not include skin cancers, of which there are an estimated 400,000 new cases annually. In Australia there are 45,000 new cases of cancer yearly and 23,000 deaths due to cancer. One Australian in 3 gets some form of serious cancer during his or her lifetime.

If cancer is diagnosed in time, the outlook is generally good. In two thirds of cases, when the cancer is first detected it is localized and amenable to surgery or radiotherapy. Of these patients in developed countries who have localized cancer, two thirds are cured. Those who are not cured have disease which has spread extensively.

The global picture shows the differences between developed and undeveloped countries. When global statistics are analyzed, two points emerge. Firstly, in the whole of the world, one tenth of deaths are due to cancer. In the West, the proportion of deaths due to cancer is more than one fifth. The types of cancer predominating in the West differ from those predominating in the rest of the world. See *geographical distribution of cancer, *incidence of cancer, *mortality from cancer, *causes of cancer.

malignant melanoma   kind of *skin cancer

mastectomy   surgical removal of breast. See *breast cancer.

malignant tumour   cancer, as distinct from *benign tumour

mammography   X-ray examination of breast. The procedure involves placing each breast, one at a time, between two flat, smooth plates, and squeezing them while the breast is X-rayed. Usually the breasts are X-rayed from the top and with an oblique or angled view and sometimes a view from the side. The squeezing does no harm but may cause discomfort. See Early Detection of Breast Cancer, under *Breast cancer.

mammaplasty   reconstructive surgery to restore breast shape after operation for *breast cancer

marijuana   dried leaves of Indian hemp, smoked or otherwise ingested for pleasurable effects. There is no proof that marijuana smoking causes cancer. However. *head and neck cancers have been reported recently in young people who have smoked marijuana. Thus, no assurances can be given that marijuana smoking is free from the risk of cancer.

meat   see *diet

medical treatment as a cause of cancer *X-rays and numerous medications are capable of causing cancer. The majority of treatments that expose patients to the risk of cancer (*chemotherapy and *radiotherapy) are those used to treat cancer itself—fighting fire with fire. Today, most physicians are only too well aware of the cancer-producing potential of such treatments. They are used in the knowledge that the risk is outweighed by the chance of benefits.

Diagnostic X-rays are not free from risk, although most modern diagnostic machines deliver smaller doses of X-rays than earlier types. X-rays can be avoided in a number of cases by using *ultrasound imaging techniques, which are free from the risk of inducing cancer. Stones can be found in gallbladders and kidneys and the moving heart can be seen pumping in pictures of reflected ultrasound waves. Most X-rays can be avoided in pregnancy, as the unborn child can be seen in the uterus by ultrasound imaging. Diseases of the stomach, bowel, bladder, pelvis and airways of the lung can be seen by *endoscopy.

The newly developed (and expensive) technique of *magnetic resonance imaging (MRI), which can be used instead of X-rays for some purposes, is free from can cancer risk.

*Radioactive iodine is given as a treatment for overactivity of the thyroid gland. This treatment has been in use for more than 40 years and has proved its safety. It is safer than an operation and the potential for causing cancer is negligible. The safety of radioiodine depends on the unique capacity of the thyroid gland to take up and use iodine. Very little radioiodine is taken up by any other tissue.

Patients who receive a transplanted kidney or other organ must take medication to suppress the immune system, which would otherwise reject the transplant. Any condition (such as *AIDS) or treatment which suppresses the immune system increases the risk of cancers, particularly *skin cancer and *lymphomas. See *immunity and cancer.

meditation ordering of thoughts, mental planning, exercise of the mind or contemplation. Meditation is akin to prayer and is a component of most religions and many personal philosophies. Some have faith in meditation as a way of combatting cancer. It is difficult to obtain valid evidence to prove or disprove the value of meditation in altering the course of cancer, but like psychological counselling and support it may prove of great value to many cancer patients. See *coping with cancer, *alternative cancer treatments.

melancholia depression of mood. See *stress, psychological factors and mental illness.

melanocyte cell in the *dermis that makes *melanin

melanoma, malignant type of *skin cancer

melanin   dark pigment of skin, hair and inside the eye, produced by *melanocytes. See *ultraviolet light, melanoma.

melphalan   medication used in cancer *chemotherapy

meningioma   benign tumour of membrane covering the brain. See *brain cancer.

MESOTHELIOMA
Mesotheliomas are cancers arising from the membranes around the lung, and occasionally the membranes lining the abdominal cavity.

Cause of Mesothelioma
Mesotheliomas are caused by inhalation of *asbestos. Of the three types of asbestos fibre—*crocidolite, *chrysotile, and *amosite—crocidolite fibres are the most dangerous.

Australia has the world's highest incidence of mesothelioma. Ten years ago mesothelioma was rare, with a yearly incidence rate averaging 1 per 2 million of the population. Since 1947 approximately 2000 cases have been documented, more than 1350 of them since 1980. To the end of 1989, 114 of these were from *Wittenoom and the incidence has jumped to a national rate of 27.9 per million for males and 3.6 for females. A rise from 200 cases a year to about 300 a year by the year 2000 is predicted. As the time from exposure to development of the disease may be 30 years or more, many new cases are anticipated before exposure to asbestos in the workplace has been

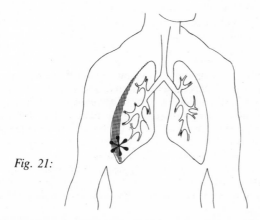

Fig. 21:

Mesothelioma. This cancer, which is caused by asbestos, grows as a plaque between the chest wall and lung.

127

controlled. In fact, the average incubation period according to Australian data is 34 years. Fifteen hundred cases occur per year in the USA.

The frequency with which exposed persons develop mesothelioma is relatively low—356 of 17,000 (2%) in 1 study. Ten to 15 per cent of cases develop without known exposure to asbestos. The chrysotile mines at *Baryulgil and *Barraba in New South Wales have not been associated with mesothelioma. Unlike *lung cancer in persons exposed to asbestos, the mesothelioma risk is not increased by smoking.

Symptoms of Mesothelioma
Patients experience either shortness of breath or pain in the chest.

Treatment of Mesothelioma
Mesothelioma is usually incurable, because the tumour is too difficult to remove by surgery. There is no effective treatment.

Prevention of Mesothelioma
It is to be hoped that the major cause of mesothelioma will soon be eliminated. Asbestos should no longer be used in buildings or electrical equipment. Workers can be exposed to fibre through demolition of buildings and removal of asbestos.

metabolic therapy   an *alternative cancer treatment, based on a special diet, which usually includes high doses of vitamins, minerals and other ingredients. It also includes a detoxification programme, usually of carrot juice, wheat grass, decaffeinated coffee and high bowel enemas of water. *Laetrile is still often included in the treatment.

Deaths have been attributed to detoxification machines which have not been cleaned properly.

metals   Heavy metals *cadmium, *chromium and *nickel, or compounds formed from them, can cause cancer.

Cadmium causes testicular tumours in rats, which can be prevented by simultaneous administration of *zinc. Cadmium has been held to cause cancer of the *prostate and *lung. Cancer of the *lung and nasal sinuses (see *head and neck cancer) occurred in nickel refinery workers until proper procedures were instituted. The active agents are in hot dusts created in the refining process.

Cancer of the *lung used to occur frequently in workers in the chromate industry, particularly in workers engaged in the manufacture of basic chromates from chrome ore, but also in the chrome-colour industry.

Exposure to these metals should by now be safely regulated in the workplace and their contribution through occupational exposure to the total number of cancers is very small.

Cadmium and nickel, as well as traces of the radioactive heavy metal *polonium-210 are present in *tobacco smoke.

metastasis   spread of cancer from the primary site to other parts of the body. A *secondary tumour, which has spread from a *primary cancer in another organ, is also referred to as a 'metastasis'.

methotrexate   medication used in cancer *chemotherapy

methylene chloride   compound causing cancer in experimental animals

methyl CCNU   trade name of medication *lomustine used in *cancer chemotherapy

microwaves   *electromagnetic radiation (like light and radio waves) between UHF (ultrahigh frequency) radio waves and heat (infrared) waves. Microwaves are used to generate heat. In medicine they are used in some types of diathermy to treat muscular and ligamentous injuries, and to induce *hyperthermia in the treatment of cancer.
   Microwave ovens have been suspected of causing cancer. There is no evidence of such an effect.

miliSievert (mSv)   unit of dosage of *radiation. 10mSv are equal to 1 rem of radiation.

mineral deficiency and cancer   Minerals are essential ingredients of a healthy diet. The average adult body contains 2–3 kg of minerals, mostly calcium and phosphorus. Of the many other minerals that are essential to life, we know something of only two—*selenium and *zinc—in the development of cancer.
   In Bulgaria, where the annual average consumption of selenium is relatively high (108 milligrams), the incidence of *breast cancer is one of the lowest. In the United States, where the annual intake of selenium is relatively low (61 miligrams), the incidence of breast cancer is high. However, this protection against cancer by a high selenium intake is not shown in all surveys.
   In a convincing study, blood samples were taken in a programme of research into high blood pressure (not cancer) in an American community in 1973. Five years later it was decided to use the blood samples for research into cancer. When the stored blood samples were tested for selenium, the average level was lower than normal in the 111 people who developed cancer **after** the blood was taken.
   Foods rich in selenium are grains, fish, meat and eggs.
   *Zinc is essential for growth. Zinc protects against cancers caused by *cadmium in experimental animals. Patients with some cancers

have been found deficient in zinc, but whether this is cause or effect is not known.

Foods rich in zinc are legumes (peas), grains, milk and dairy products, meat, poultry, crustaceans and sea fish.

mineral oils   cause of *skin cancer in persons engaged in the oil, *shale oil and associated motor industries. Oils deliver *polycylic hydrocarbons to the skin, but to cause cancer, exposure must be prolonged. In a recent Swedish study of 792 machine tool operators, 7 of the turners, each of whom used cutting fluids containing mineral oils, but none of the grinders, had *squamous cell cancer of the *scrotum.

mitomycin   medication used in cancer *chemotherapy

Mitomycin C   trade name of *mitomycin

mitoxantrone   medication used in cancer *chemotherapy

mole   any dark or pigmented spot or malformation on the skin. Moles usually arise after birth and change little thereafter. *Skin cancer may develop in some pigmented moles. The term *naevus is used interchangeably with 'mole'.

Mongolism   see *Down's syndrome

monoclonal antibodies   antibodies made in the laboratory by growing selected cells which produce antibody having the desired characteristics. See *immunity and cancer.

Montagnier, Luc   contemporary French virologist, co-discoverer with *Gallo of *HIV as the cause of *AIDS

morphine   major *pain-relieving narcotic used in medicine. Morphine and many other narcotics are prepared from the sap of the opium poppy *Papaver somniferum*. Morphine has various side effects, including loss of appetite and constipation. In overdose it causes *nausea, depression of respiration and loss of consciousness. Morphine can be given by mouth and by various types of injection, including slow infusion around the spinal cord.

The general principle for use of morphine and related medications for the relief of pain in cancer patients is that adequate doses should be given to anticipate and control pain. *Addiction is often a concern of cancer patients, who should generally be reassured that it is not a serious problem, for two reasons: addiction does not occur readily in persons who have narcotics for the relief of severe pain; and dependence on morphine is a small price to pay, when considered in the light of intractable pain, which otherwise makes life a misery.

MORTALITY FROM CANCER

Table 10: Mortality from different types of cancer

Number of persons in each 100,000 of the population who die from
particular cancers each year

Type	Males	Females
Breast		25
Lung	52	16
Large Bowel	28	22
Prostate	22	
Melanoma	5	4
Stomach	12	6
Lymphoma	8	6
Leukaemia	8	6
Cervix		3
Uterus (Endometrium)		4
Ovary		8
Pancreas	9	9
Kidney and ureters	5	2
Bladder	6	2
Brain	7	4
Multiple myeloma	3	3
All Sites	193	136

These 1987 figures from the South Australian Cancer Registry are
representative of most Western societies

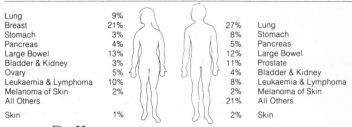

Lung	9%	27%	Lung
Breast	21%	8%	Stomach
Stomach	3%	5%	Pancreas
Pancreas	4%	12%	Large Bowel
Large Bowel	13%	11%	Prostate
Bladder & Kidney	3%	4%	Bladder & Kidney
Ovary	5%	8%	Leukaemia & Lymphoma
Leukaemia & Lymphoma	10%	2%	Melanoma of Skin
Melanoma of Skin	2%	21%	All Others
All Others			
Skin	1%	2%	Skin

Fig. 22:

*Relative mortality from different types of cancer. These figures
show the relative contribution of different cancers to total deaths
caused by cancer, in females and males. The figures were
compiled from US and Australian data and represent typical
Western statistics. By comparing these figures it can be seen that
some cancers are responsible for a porportion of deaths exceeding
their relative frequency, as shown in Fig. 45.* See also *magnitude
of the cancer problem, incidence of cancer.

mouth cancer   see *head and neck cancer

multiple myeloma   a type of cancer of cells of the immune system, affecting bones. See *bone cancer.

mustard gas   compound used in chemical warfare that may cause cancer. In World Wars I and II mustard gas was observed to cause wasting of lymphoid tissues and reduction in size of tumours. After World War II compounds related to mustard gas were tested for anti-cancer activity. Some of these compounds became the earliest effective medications for cancer *chemotherapy.

mutation   change in *DNA, amounting to falsification of the genetic blueprint. A mutation is inherited by all progeny of the cell in which it has occurred. Most mutations are harmful to cells and some result in the loss of control of growth that amounts to cancer. See *nature of cancer.

N

naevus malformed spot on the skin, usually pigmented, arising after birth and usually changing little. Skin cancer can develop in some pigmented naevi. The term 'naevus' is used interchangeably with '*mole'. See *dysplastic naevus syndrome.

Nagasaki Japanese city destroyed by an atomic bomb in World War II on August 9th, 1945. See *atomic bombs and nuclear reactors.

names of cancers Cancers are divided into the *carcinomas (from the Greek *karkinos*, crab, and *karkinoma*, ulcer) and the *sarcomas (Greek *sarx, sarkos*, flesh). The term 'karkinoma' was used by the Greek physician Hippocrates (ca. 469–370 BC) for cancer.

Carcinomas are derived from *epithelium. Epithelial cells line parts of the body that come into contact with the outside world and also form glands which make products for export around the body. Examples of epithelial lining cells are those lining the gut and cells of the skin. Examples of epithelial glands are the pancreas and liver. Tumours of all of these are called carcinomas.

Cancers of the supporting and connective tissues are called sarcomas. An example is *osteosarcoma, a cancer of bone.

This distinction was made by the early pathologists, but nowadays has little practical importance.

The original tumour is called the *primary tumour. Tumours in distant sites that have spread by blood or lymph vessels are called *secondary tumours or *metastases (from Greek '*methistemi*', change). Secondary tumours usually have characteristics of the primary, but may show more malignant features.

naphthylamine *aniline dye, capable of causing *bladder cancer, particularly in workers in the dye industry

nasopharyngeal carcinoma relatively common in Southern China but very rare in Europeans, is a cancer of the back of the nasal cavity. Two factors are at work to cause this cancer, infection with the *Epstein-Barr virus (as in *Burkitt's lymphoma) and *nitrosamines. The *nitrosamines come from salted fish, a staple diet for many in communities at high risk for nasopharyngeal carcinoma. Eating salted fish in childhood increases the risk by 20 to 30 times. The part played by nitrosamines has been confirmed by showing that these compounds cause nasopharyngeal cancers when given to rats.

Natulan trade name of *procarbazine, medication used in cancer *chemotherapy

NATURE OF CANCER

Cancer has been known and feared since antiquity, but the nature of cancer could only be understood when *cells were recognized. Much of the modern understanding of cancer began with the German pathologist *Virchow, who argued that the basis of cancer is an abnormality of growth of cells.

Cancers are tissues that grow abnormally to the detriment of their hosts. The key to understanding cancer is understanding growth and the abnormalities of growth that lead to cancer.

Growth starts with fertilization of the ovum and reaches a steady state when adult size is reached. The new individual grows by multiplication of cells. The first cell divides to produce two daughter cells; daughter cells divide again; and so on. The adult is made up of billions of cells, all descended from the first and all having developed special characteristics. The miracle of growth is essentially the production of cells in the right number and at the right place. Furthermore, as the individual grows, groups of cells develop different functions.

To make each part of the body, cells become specialized by a process called *differentiation. Certain cells begin to differentiate, from very early in life, so that the newly developing body has head and toes, a front and a back and so on. The symmetry of the body is itself a miracle, each hand, for example, growing as a mirror image of the other, without any direct communication during growth.

Growth from a single cell to a perfectly formed baby is occasionally disturbed by infections or by medications taken by the mother. For example, the drug thalidomide resulted in failure of growth of limbs. This failure to grow is the opposite of cancer, in which growth continues without ever stopping. These two extreme examples raise the question: 'How does a cell know when to divide and when to stop dividing?'

The strictly regulated growth pattern of normal tissues is lost in cancer. When a cell becomes malignant, its daughter cells do not differentiate fully. They keep on dividing and they live longer. The net result is steady, never-ending increase in the number of cells.

Many questions posed by cancer are fundamental biological questions. For example, how is growth controlled, from a single cell at conception to an inconceivably complex organism of a vast number of cells? How does the body stop growing? How do cells differentiate into specialized cells for different organs, e.g. skin, blood, brain? How does a cell 'know' when to multiply and when to stop? How is differentiation, i.e. the development of specialized characteristics, controlled?

The answer to these questions lies in the interplay between the hereditary blueprint of a cell, its *DNA, and chemical messages from other cells. This interplay is disrupted in cancer. Every cell inherits a

134

full copy of the DNA blueprint which specifies how each part of the cell is made and how it should respond to these messages from other cells. For each cell to take its place according to the master plan of the body, it must respond appropriately, both to its neighbours and to the needs of the whole body.

The basic fault in a cancer cell lies in changes in its DNA. Particular changes in the DNA blueprint allow a cell to escape the control exerted by chemical messages from its neighbours. When such a cell arises, all of its progeny inherit the change and as a result, they also escape normal controls on growth.

Even in adulthood growth takes place to replace aged and damaged cells. In healthy adults, millions of cells in the skin, bowel, blood and other organs die each day. They body replaces the lost cells at precisely the same rate as they are lost. The highly accurate maintenance of the status quo depends upon chemical regulation of growth.

There are some obvious differences between growth from conception to birth and growth in adulthood, when only worn out cells are replaced. Most cancers occur in adulthood and they arise in groups of cells responsible for this replacement process.

Growth Factors and Hormones

Growth factors and hormones are the chemical messages which control growth. Cells are constantly giving and receiving messages that influence each other to grow or to remain quiescent. *Growth factors and *hormones are natural chemical substances that stimulate cells to divide, giving rise to two cells where there was formerly one.

Growth factors are made in many types of cell throughout the body. They act at short range and many types of growth factor last for a short time, soon being degraded. In this way they only act on cells in the neighbourhood and do not travel far in the blood. Cells also send messages to each other when they touch.

Growth factors bind to *receptors on the surface of target cells, initiating biochemical chain reactions that result in growth. Now that the structure of many growth factors is known, it is possible to produce them in the laboratory, and some have become available for clinical use.

Hormones also influence the growth of many classes of cells. Hormones are made in one organ and circulate around the body. Sex hormones and growth hormone are examples. Hormones tell all cells of the needs of the whole body, in contrast to growth factors, which tell neighbouring cells of the requirements of the organ or tissue.

Repair of a cut in the skin illustrates the action of growth factors. The cut deprives certain deeper cells of their covering layer. These cells respond by making growth factor that stimulates outer skin cells to divide. When the defect is repaired, growth factor production

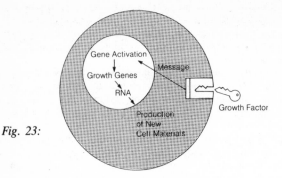

Fig. 23:

Chemical messenger and receptor. Chemical messengers, including growth factors, fit their own receptors, but not the receptors for other chemical messengers. Binding to the receptor sets off a chain of chemical reactions that results in production of cell materials for growth. In the illustration, the reaction causes activation of certain genes *whose* protein *products are necessary for growth. Activation of a gene involves transcription in the* nucleus *of an* RNA *template or set of instructions on how protein is to be made. The new materials for growth are then made in the* cytoplasm. *This illustration shows the fundamental chain of events necessary for growth — initiation by a chemical messenger such as a* growth factor *and activation of particular genes, so that the information encoded in those genes can be read out in the form of an* RNA transcript *that is then used by the cellular machinery to produce the required protein. Abnormalities of this sequence, usually resulting from faulty* DNA, *are the basis of malignant growth.*

ceases and the outer skin cells stop dividing. A superficial wound heals without trace.

Haemorrhage offers another illustration. When a person suffers haemorrhage, billions of red blood cells are lost. When blood is lost the replacement mechanisms are switched into top gear, restoring the blood volume to normal as quickly as possible. The deficiency of red cells is detected by sensors in the kidneys, which respond by producing the red cell growth factor *erythropoietin. Erythropoietin stimulates the *bone marrow to produce red cells. When normal blood levels are reached, the rate of replacement returns to normal. **The growth of cancer cells proceeds without these normal controls by growth factors and hormones.**

Stem Cells

The replacement of worn out or damaged cells is the job of certain cells, called *stem cells, that are capable of frequent division.

The stem cells are not working cells; that is, they do not carry out the special job of the tissue. They exist to replace the normal working cells that die.

Normally a stem cell divides to produce one daughter cell that leaves the home base and one that takes the place of the parent cell. It is rather like what has to happen in a farming family. When the parents go, one son stays on the farm and the other children have to leave home.

Daughters of stem cells that leave home base differentiate into specialized cells that lose their capacity to divide, and have a limited life.

In the skin, stem cells lie on a basement membrane. These are the only cells in the outer layer of normal skin—the epidermis—which can proliferate. When a stem cell divides, only one of the daughter cells can stay on this basement membrane. This one replaces its parent and retains the capacity to divide. The other daughter cell progresses towards the exterior, as new cells are formed beneath it, and undergoes *differentiation to make the waterproof materials that seal the surface. As it is pushed towards the surface, the cell dies, dries out and eventually flakes off. Daughter cells lose their capacity to divide when they leave the basement membrane.

The tissue under the epidermis, the dermis, produces substances that regulate the growth of epidermal cells.

In a wart, a benign tumour of the skin, this very closely controlled limitation of division to the innermost layer of cells is lost. When a stem cell in a wart gives rise to two daughter cells, both of them may retain the capacity to divide.

In a skin cancer, dividing cells can be seen several layers out from the basement membrane.

In normal tissues, the proportion of cells undergoing division is relatively small. The proportion of dividing cells is frequently quite large in a cancer.

Differentiation

Differentiation is specialization for highly technical jobs. Cells may undergo remarkable changes when they differentiate. A nerve cell has a very long extension, like a telephone line for transmitting the nerve signal. A long, thin muscle cell contracts when it receives an impulse from its nerve. A liver cell makes raw materials and specialized compounds which it exports all round the body via the blood.

In tissues where cells are replaced at a high rate, such as skin, bowel and blood, the differentiated working cells live only for a short time. In some highly specialized tissues, such as muscle and brain, there are few stem cells or none at all and the differentiated cells have

Nature of cancer

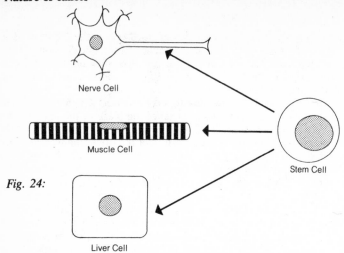

Fig. 24:

Nerve Cell

Muscle Cell

Stem Cell

Liver Cell

Examples of differentiation. All cells have the information in their DNA *blueprint to make structures required by specialised cells. An undifferentiated cell illustrated on the right could become a nerve cell, a muscle cell or a liver cell if subjected to the appropriate influences during development. Differentiation is brought about by activation of a particular set of genes, so that the cell can produce the necessary structures for specialised function.* See Fig. 23.

a very long life. When these highly specialized cells are lost there are no cells from which a new population may grow. Since cancers arise in stem cells, tumours of nerve cells and muscle are very rare. (Cancers of the adult *brain arise from supporting cells, rather than nerve cells.)

Once a normal cell has become specialized it loses the capacity to divide. By contrast, even though imperfect specialization has occurred in a cancer cell, it may not lose its capacity to divide. As a result, a relatively large proportion of cells in a cancer have the capacity to contribute to its growth.

Not only can cancer cells continue to reproduce, but they can also reproduce into old age. Once born, cancer cells often have a long lifespan. Imagine the increase of a human population if nobody died. Even worse, imagine if people did not stop having children in later life. **A population increases if more are born than die. This simple fact is at the root of the cancer problem.**

Characteristics of Cancers

The characteristics of cancers are the result of the properties of the cancer cells themselves (Table 11).

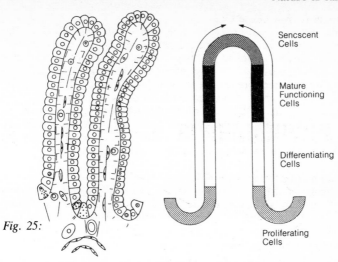

Fig. 25:

Intestinal mucous membrane. This is a cross section of two finger-like fronds in the lining of the intestine (left). The stem cells at the bottom are multiplying continuously. Daughter cells that move towards the apex of the frond do not multiply. As they move upwards they differentiate. The process is illustrated schematically on the right, showing four zones: proliferation (containing the stem cells), differentiation, mature functioning cells and senescent cells that will soon drop off. Normally only the stem cells multiply. Tissue beneath the membrane on which the lining cells sit contains blood and lymph vessels, and cells which produce growth factors that stimulate stem cells based on the membrane. Growth in adult life is normally confined to replacement of lost and worn out cells. Cancer arises when one of the stem cells develops an abnormality of growth, such that it multiples without control, producing abnormal cells that themselves continue to multiply.

Table 11: Characteristics of cancers

1	Each cancer arises from a single stem cell
2	Cancers never stop growing
3	Cancers spread directly and by vessels
4	Cancers cause damage by invading tissues and producing harmful substances

139

Nature of cancer

Origin from a Single Cell

Like its host, a cancer also starts in a single cell. Out of all the cells subjected to carcinogenic influences, one emerges with all the characteristics needed to found a cancer dynasty. Each of its progeny inherits the the parent cell's disregard for its neighbours and its host. Using modern techniques, the unique characteristics of the original malignant cell can be demonstrated in all of its descendants.

Cancer is actually hundreds of diseases which have the same basic disorder of growth control. Because each cancer develops from an individual cell, no two cancers are exactly alike, but cancers arising from a particular tissue have a similar pattern of behaviour.

Cancers arise from Stem Cells

Damage to the genetic blueprint of a cell that is destined to die hardly matters, so long as it is replaced by a normal cell. Damage to the blueprint of a stem cell is another matter, because its progeny can inherit a damaged blueprint. In this way, the damaging effect of a carcinogen can be passed on by a dividing stem cell to all of its progeny.

We know that the primary damage caused by exposure to a carcinogenic agent can occur years before the cancer develops. This primary damage must occur in a stem cell. Secondary damage, occurring at a later date, sets the damaged stem cell dividing out of control. No other mechanism explains the long memory of the primary damage. Only the stem cells can perpetuate the primary genetic damage over the years of the lead time between the insult, such as exposure to an *atomic bomb, and the development of cancer.

Cancers do not stop Growing

Cancer cells do not develop to maturity, work responsibly or grow old and die like normal cells. Cancer cells have the capacity to multiply indefinitely; that is, they are potentially immortal. Normal cells are not immortal. If given the chance to multiply without restraint, with ample nutrition and the necessary growth factors, normal stem cells ultimately stop dividing. There is an inbuilt limit to the number of divisions they can undergo. That is why creatures have a limited life.

The antisocial activity of individual cancer cells is reminiscent of growth of single-cell organisms, like amoebae and bacteria, which arose early in evolution. The preoccupation of single-cell organisms is competition for nourishment. Unlike most single-cell parasites, however, the cancer cell dies when it kills the host, whereas mechanisms have evolved in many parasites for more peaceful coexistence and for survival in a dormant form should the nourishment be exhausted.

A distinction is made between *benign and *malignant tumours, because of differences in behaviour. Most malignant tumours have a

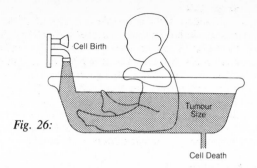

Fig. 26:

Why cancers get bigger. Tumours grow if the number of cells formed exceeds the number dying. Here the production of new cells (the tap) is greater than cell death (the drain), threatening a disaster. Proliferation by itself is not enough for increase in tumour size, if the cells have a very short lifespan (equivalent to a large drain). Tumour cells often live for a very long time.

benign counterpart. Benign tumours are very important for understanding the development of malignant tumours, as they sometimes represent a stage in the development of a malignant tumour. Bowel cancers frequently develop from within benign tumours.

The major distinction is that benign tumours do not spread by the blood or *lymph streams. Each kind of tumour still represents a disorder of growth. A tumour is considered to be benign if it grows slowly, does not seriously invade surrounding tissues, and does not spread to distant parts of the body. A benign tumour of skin or bowel does not grow down into underlying tissues. A benign tumour can be cured by simply removing it. A malignant tumour will spread to other organs at some time. Sometimes malignant tumours have already spread by the time they are removed.

Cancers do their damage in two ways, (1) by simply existing, occupying space to the detriment of the normal tissues they invade and (2) by interfering in some way with the activities of the normal cells. This interference usually results from substances released by the cancer cells, which interfere with the chemical processes of the normal cells.

*Metastasis occurs frequently to some tissues, and rarely to others. Each type of tumour has a common pattern of direct spread and metastasis. Spread to bones may cause fractures and pain. Spread to the brain may cause paralysis and disturbances of mental function.

Normal Cells in Cancer Tissues

Cancers resemble cuckoos and other parasites. The young cuckoo survives because an ingenuous bird has been tricked into providing

141

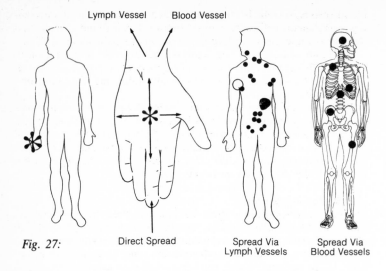

Lymph Vessel   Blood Vessel

Fig. 27:   Direct Spread   Spread Via Lymph Vessels   Spread Via Blood Vessels

Spread of cancer. Cancers spread (a) directly into the body from the part in which they arise (b) by blood vessels and (c) by lymphatic vessels.

Fig. 28:

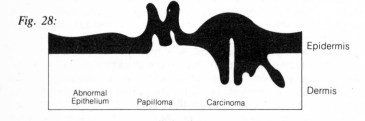

Epidermis

Abnormal Epithelium   Papilloma   Carcinoma

Dermis

Stages in the development of a tumour. In the skin, cancer develops frequently in an area where growth of cells is abnormal ('abnormal epithelium'). A benign tumour is often like a wart (a 'papilloma'). Sometimes a fern-like growth pattern may form a polyp, particularly in the bowel. Benign skin tumours do not spread into the underlying epidermis. The malignant tumour ('carcinoma') starts to invade the deeper tissues.

board and lodging. A cancer also survives by tricking the host into providing nourishment. For a cancer to be successful, it must entice cells from neighbouring normal blood vessels to grow into the tumour. The cancer cells do this by making growth factors for host

142

blood vessels, so-called *angiogenesis factors. One of the characteristics a malignant cell must acquire before it can found a malignant dynasty is the capacity to lure blood vessels to grow along with it.

One kind of cancer—*leukaemia—does not rely on angiogenesis factors. Leukaemic cells are the malignant counterpart of normal circulating blood cells. They exist singly, obtaining their nutrition directly from the blood.

The early tumour is relatively well ordered, bearing many resemblances to its tissue of origin. In its later stages, for example in metastases, the pathologist sees bizarre cells, which are irregular in size and shape. These irregular cells usually have abnormalities of chromosomes, reflecting the tendency for cancer cells to undergo further damage to DNA as the cancer gets older.

Evolution in Cancers

Cancers evolve during their lifespan and become progressively more aggressive. This process results from successive accidental changes to the blueprint in individual cancer cells, permitting progressively stronger growth. The process is the same as Darwinian evolution. Weak cells die, strong cells grow more vigorously. Changes to the blueprint, known as *mutations, frequently permit individual cancer cells to escape from *radiotherapy or *chemotherapy. A cell that resists treatment can found a treatment-resistant *clone.

When treatment-resistant tumours are examined microscopically, they are often much more irregular and disorderly than the original cancer, because of unrestrained growth. For example, cells in these tumours do not respect their neighbours and push against them.

Cancer Results from Falsification of the Cell's Blueprint

Clearly there is a blueprint of the whole organism in each cell, and each cell is programmed to fulfil its destiny in the master plan. The blueprint for each type of cell, the master plan of *differentiation for all of the cells and their place in the tissues, is contained in the first cell, the new individual that arises when the father's sperm joins the mother's ovum. This blueprint is written in material called *DNA in a chemical language known as the *genetic code. When a cell divides, every daughter cell receives a copy of the DNA blueprint. This DNA blueprint for life contains a complete set of instructions on how to build any type of cell and therefore how to build an individual.

The DNA chemical language uses an alphabet of only four chemical letters and all words contain three letters. A chemical sentence, amounting to a unit of information in the blueprint is called a *gene. Each gene is the specification for manufacture of a *protein product. The cell's blueprint is not a flat picture, but a set of long strings of genes, called *chromosomes.

The blueprint of the new individual is a combination of genes derived from the parents. To make its essential tools and structural

Nature of cancer

materials, the cell turns to its genes to obtain the necessary information. Each gene is a set of instructions for making a part of a cell in a material called *protein. Proteins are the essential material for beams and pillars (cell skeleton), moving parts (muscle) and chemical tools (*enzymes) of the cell. Having the necessary proteins, the cell can make and do everything it is called upon to do. For example it can generate energy by burning sugars and fats and use this energy for manufacture of all the products it needs for itself and for export. It can use this energy to move, take in food and raw materials, contract (if it is a muscle cell) or make an electric current (if it is a nerve cell). Besides protein, it can make other types of material like *fats and *carbohydrates.

Each cell uses only a fraction of the genes it possesses. To differentiate, cells use different genes. In this way cells add new equipment to the basic model. The pattern of genes that is needed by each type of specialised cell is also written in the blueprint.

During the development of the baby in the uterus, cells destined to become nerve, muscle or skin cells, for example, use the pertinent genes to make the proteins peculiar to each of these types of cells. Knowing the nature of genes, we can begin to understand the process of differentiation. Differentiation is really selection of particular sets of genes from which the cell shall make proteins.

The rules of the *genetic code are as follows:
(1) The alphabet contains only four chemical letters, which can be used in any order.

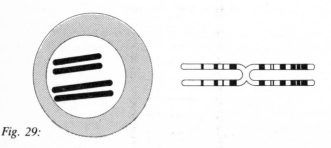

Fig. 29:

Chromosomes. Chromosomes are long paired threads of DNA. *The threads are normally tightly wound around a core like fishing line to enable them to fit into the nucleus. Each human cell contains 22 matching pairs of general chromosomes, and another pair of sex chromosomes. The chromosomes shown on the left represent two pairs in a resting cell. The chromosome on the right is shown as chromosomes are usually seen, having doubled themselves immediately before division. When stained each chromosome can be recognised by a distinctive pattern of bands.*

(2) Each word contains only three letters.
(3) Sentences can be short or very long.
(4) There is no punctuation between words, only at the end of sentences.
(5) The same code is used for every living creature.

The whole book, or *genome, is written in three-letter words, using only the four chemical letters. The genes are sentences, the chromosomes are chapters and the book contains many chapters. Each chromosome contains thousands of genes. Individual genes always occupy the same place on the same chromosome.

This seemingly simple *genetic code permits storage of vast quantities of information. Decoded, the whole blueprint written in legible letters would fill a thousand telephone directories.

Just as the code for all forms of life is universal, so also is the nature of *protein, the product of the code. Proteins are the basic structural materials from which all plants and animals are built.

A chromosome has two spiral strands of DNA, a master strand and a backup strand. The backup strand is a complementary copy, not a direct copy. Each letter of the master or working strand matches its complementary letter on the backup strand. A is complementary to T, and G is complementary to C.

To understand the shape of DNA, imagine a ladder, then twist it like a strap of liquorice into a spiral. A twisted ladder would form two spirals joined by rungs. DNA looks just like this.

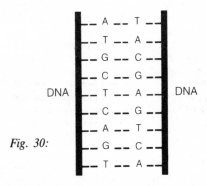

Fig. 30:

Untwisted DNA. If the double helix of DNA is untwisted, it has the shape of a ladder. The rungs of the ladder are equivalent to the complementary matching chemical letters of the genetic code and the sides are the chemical backbones of the two strands of DNA. Compare this with DNA in the normal form of a double helix, shown in Fig. 15.

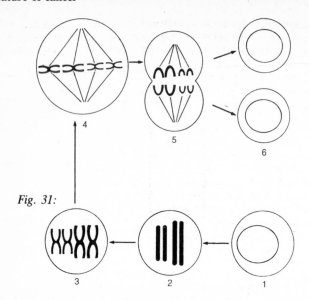

Fig. 31:

Chromosomes during cell division. This illustration depicts the events in an imaginary species which has two pairs of chromosomes (humans have 23 pairs). In a cell which will divide (1), the chromosomes condense and become visible (2). Next, each chromosome is copied, giving a double quota (3). The chromosomes then line up across a central plane of the cell and become attached to fibres radiating from each pole of the cell (4). The fibres pull one copy of each chromosome to each half (5). After the two halves split apart, there are two daughter cells (6). The end result of this process is that each daughter cell gets a complete copy of the individual's DNA blueprint. The process by which the double helix of each chromosome is doubled is illustrated in Fig. 32.

Conversely, if DNA is straightened out or untwisted it looks like a ladder (Fig. 30). The two long supports are the chemical backbone and the rungs are made of the paired matching letters. There are only two types of rung, A-T (or T-A) and G-C (or C-G).

The nuclei of human cells contain 23 pairs of chromosomes. Figure 29 shows a cell with only two pairs of chromosomes. Before cell division each chromosome is doubled. Each daughter receives one copy of each chromosome present in its parent.

For each daughter cell arising by cell division to have a copy of the blueprint, there must be a mechanism for copying DNA. In principle,

146

the copying process is simple. One letter of the code is matched with its complementary letter (Fig 32). To divide, the spirals in the double helix separate—the ladder splits down the middle, the rungs coming apart where the letters join. Then a complementary half ladder is made according to the pattern of each single half. The result is two identical double helices.

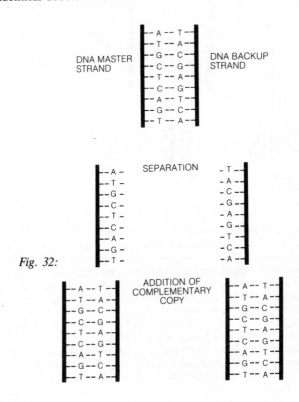

Fig. 32:

Replication of double-stranded DNA. Each chromosome has two strands of DNA, but uses only one strand as the master code. Each letter of the code is matched on the complementary strand by its complementary letter. A always matches T, and G always matches C. To make a copy, the cell separates the strands and uses each separate strand as a template. The end result is identical double-stranded chromosomes. By this means each daughter cell can be provided with an exact and complete blueprint of the whole individual.

Nature of cancer

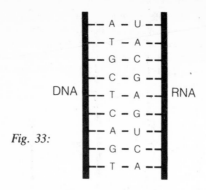

Fig. 33:

Transcribing DNA into RNA. The first step in making a protein is to get a copy of the instructions written in DNA code, in the form of an RNA printout. Like DNA, RNA has an alphabet of four letters, but uses the letters A, U, G and C. A in RNA matches T in DNA, G matches C.

Translating the Genetic Code
When a gene is activated (see Fig 33), a transcript of it is made in *RNA, a linear printout of the gene in similar but not identical chemical letters. The *amino acids, building blocks of protein, are joined end to end in the order specified in the RNA printout (Fig 34). The shape of the protein depends entirely on the amino acids and on the order in which they occur. Proteins may be long and straight, globular, tangled skeins, flat sheets or tubes. The machinery is complex, but the principle is simple.

Relevance of the Genetic Code to Cancer
A fault in the code results in faulty products. When the code is falsified, the cells are not constructed properly and do not work properly. Particular faulty products cause cancerous behaviour of cells.

How the Genetic Blueprint may be Falsified
The errors in the blueprint that result in cancer can be caused by *chemicals, *radiations and *viruses.
Virtually any disturbance of the DNA constitutes a *mutation. Change to a sentence, or even to a single letter, may be enough to cause cancer. If damaged DNA is not repaired, the damaged parts are copied exactly when the cell divides. Therefore each member of the clone inherits whatever advantage or disadvantage the mutation has given the ancestor.

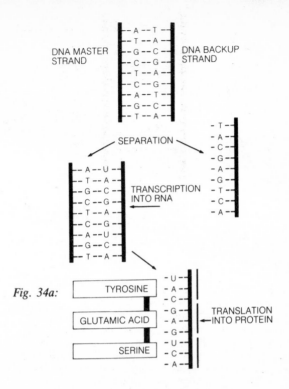

Fig. 34a:

Production of protein: translating the genetic code. Protein is made on a template of RNA. The information for making a protein is written in DNA code. To use the code, the cell must make a printout of this information, in a slightly different chemical language called RNA. This sequence shows that when a gene is activated so that the cell can make specific protein encoded by the gene, the backup strand separates from the master strand. Then an RNA copy is made, matching each letter in the DNA with the complementary RNA letter. A of DNA is matched by U of RNA, G matches C and T of DNA is matched by A of RNA. Each three-letter word in the RNA designates an amino acid. The process of joining the amino acids is illustrated in Fig. 34b.

Chemical carcinogens cause cancer by binding to DNA and setting up chemical reactions. The change resulting from such reactions can be to a single letter in the code, or to long stretches of DNA. X-rays, on the other hand, act to knock out one or more letters.

Nature of cancer

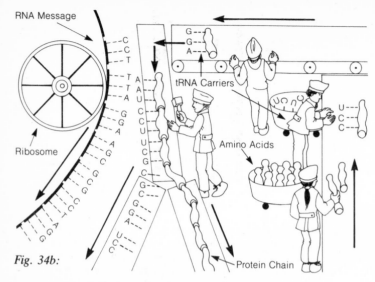

Fig. 34b:

Manufacture of protein using the RNA printout. Protein is made by joining chemical building blocks called amino acids together top to tail. This picture illustrates the mechanics of hooking together the amino acids in the sequence prescribed by the RNA printout. In the first step, a carrier is fitted to the amino acid. Each type of amino acid has a carrier. An image of the RNA code on the back of the carrier matches exactly one of the three-letter words of RNA. Amino acids attached to carriers are then matched to each three-letter word of the RNA message in turn. The message acts as a template while the amino acid is hooked on to the preceding one. The carriers are detached from the elongating amino acid chain.

Viruses cause malignant change by putting one or more of their own genes into the chromosomes of the host. Viral genes disrupt cellular function in two ways. One way is to cause overactivity of the host's genes. Another way is to put one of its own growth genes, called an *oncogene, into the chromosome. This leads to production of a protein that upsets the cell's growth. Viral oncogenes are actually faulty copies of normal genes used for growth.

In the laboratory, viral oncogenes can be isolated and inserted into cells in culture. The recipient cells acquire malignant characteristics. Oncogenes turn nonmalignant cells into cancer cells.

Oncogenes are comparable to computer 'viruses', which 'infect' computer programmes and lead to uncontrolled activity. A computer

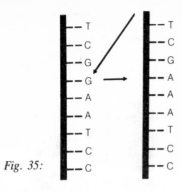

Mutation affecting a single letter of the code. A mutation is essentially any form of damage or disarrangement of a cell's DNA. The simplest mutation is a change in only one of the letters of DNA. The damaged DNA letter G (guanine) is incorrectly repaired, resulting in a change to A (adenine). The new three-letter word specifies a different amino acid and the protein encoded by this segment of DNA is changed. Growth will be affected if the abnormal protein is involved in growth processes.

virus can cause any part of the host's programme to be deleted or changed, causing 'mutations' in the software. Computer viruses can also cause parts of the programme to be copied—a kind of 'malignant growth' of software.

An oncogene may turn on genes that are not normally used by particular types of cell. For example, a cell from the bowel may be perverted to make a hormone that should only be made elsewhere in the body. Such disturbances contribute to the illness caused by the cancer.

Cells have more sophisticated defences against falsification of their genetic programmes than computers. Cells copy the genetic blueprint with astonishing accuracy and rectify errors they may make during copying. However, if an error is not corrected, it is copied faithfully and handed on to all the cell's descendants. Some rare inherited cancer syndromes are due to the absence of mechanisms for repairing damage to DNA. Cancer cells themselves become less efficient at correcting errors during copying, with the result that cells arise from time to time that are more malignant than their ancestors.

A malignant change can also be started by a tangle in two chromosomes. When a cell divides, the long skeins of DNA destined for the daughter cells are normally pulled into each new cell. Rarely, the strands tangle, break and rejoin at the wrong places, a process called

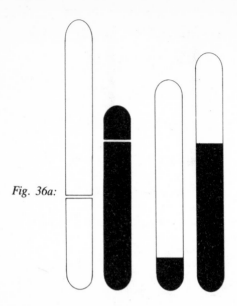

Fig. 36a:

Chromosomal translocation. A translocation is a displacement of one or more lengths of DNA from their proper position in the chromosomes. In the illustration, breaks have occurred in two chromosomes (left). The bottom end of the light-coloured chromosome has joined the bottom end of the darker chromosome and the two top ends have joined. This results in parts of chromosomes coming together in a new arrangement, and also in the parts being joined in the wrong direction. The main trouble from translocations occurs at the points where chromosomes break and wrongly rejoin. Sentences become disjointed and their sense is altered.

*translocation (Fig 36). It is like breaking two sentences and joining the wrong segments together .

Genetic Errors Accumulate in Cancers

Descendants of the original malignant cell become increasingly susceptible to further changes in the DNA. This may result from faults in the mechanism for copying DNA. Ultimately a cell will arise which is even more malignant than its predecessors. The descendants of this new cell form a new dynasty of cancer cells, a subclone which can outgrow the original *clone.

While the cancer exists, this process never stops. The cancer becomes more and more malignant.

TAKE THE MONEY TO THE BANK

ON THURSDAY.

Collect Friday's rubbish

and throw it out.

TAKE THE MONEY TO THE BANK

and throw it out.

Fig 36b:

Collect Friday's rubbish ON THURSDAY.

A verbal translocation. If chromosomal strands tangle they may break and rejoin at the wrong breakpoints. The result is called translocation. In the analogy of a chromosome as a chapter and a gene as a sentence, we see here the text torn in mid sentence and the wrong halves rejoined, making two nonsense sentences.

nasal cavity cancer   see *head and neck cancer

nausea   disagreeable sensation in the abdomen that precedes vomiting. Like *pain, nausea is strongly influenced by psychological factors and can be evaluated only by the patient. Among the many causes of nausea are abdominal disease, abnormal chemical balance in the blood, disturbance of the balance organ of the inner ear, drugs and raised pressure inside the skull.
Nausea is relieved if the cause can be treated. Otherwise, medications can be given to relieve the symptom.

neurofibromatosis   or von Recklinghausen's syndrome (described by *von Recklinghausen in 1882) is a relatively common disorder, occurring in 1 in 3000 persons, characterised by pigmented skin patches together with tumours of the skin. In this condition *benign fibrous tumours of nerves develop. There is a 50% risk for each offspring of an affected patient to have patches of pigmentation or skin tumours. Persons who have this condition are prone to develop certain rare malignancies, such as *meningiomas or tumours of nerves.

nickel   metallic element. Nickel refinery workers used to develop cancers of the *lung and nasal sinuses (*see head and neck cancer) until measures were take to protect workers from heated dusts arising from the refining process. See *metals.

nicotine   addictive substance in *tobacco. A nerve stimulant.

nitrates, nitrites   chemical compounds incorporating nitrogen oxides. See *nitrosamines.

nitrogen oxides   gases formed during combustion of petroleum and other fuels, that can be used to form carcinogenic *nitrosamines. Nitrogen oxides interact with hydrocarbons to form *ozone, which blocks *ultraviolet light. See *air pollution.

4-nitrophenyl   chemical of the *aromatic amine class, found in *tobacco smoke. See *occupation and cancer.

nitrosamines   compounds formed in the body by interaction of nit rates or nitrites with various abundant compounds in food (called amines), under acid conditions such as exist in the stomach. Nitrates and nitrites are added to pork products (ham, fritz, salami, sausage etc) to prevent them becoming rancid and to give them a red colour. Some vegetables, such as beets, radishes, spinach and lettuce are rich in nitrates.
   Nitrosamines cause cancer in experimental animals and are thought likely to be a cause of cancer, particularly of the *stomach and of *nasopharyngeal cancer in humans living in poor parts of the world. The risk to humans from nitrosamines in food appears to be miniscule if they eat fresh food. The risk can be diminished further by eating foods that contain *vitamins C and E, and by avoiding foods to which nitrites or nitrates are added (eg cured meats and sausages).
   Nitrosamines are formed during the processing of *tobacco. They are therefore important not only in tobacco which is smoked, but in snuff and chewing tobacco.

Novantrone   trade name of *mitoxantrone, medication used in *chemotherapy

nuclear accident   see *atomic bombs and nuclear reactors

nucleotides   chemical name for units that make up *DNA acting as letters in the *genetic code. Also known as 'bases'.

nucleus   part of all *cells, containing the genetic material *DNA and acting as the cells' control centre. The nucleus is usually a spherical body in the middle of the cell.

Nutrasweet   see *aspartame

O

obesity overweight, a factor in susceptibility to cancer. See *diet and cancer, *breast, *ovary, *uterus cancer.

occupation and cancer Cancer of the *scrotum, a very rare type of cancer today, was the first industrial cancer to be recognised. Occurring in chimney sweeps, its cause was *soot. It is found occasionally today in automatic lathe operators, workers in petroleum refineries and the shale oil industry, and is due in these cases to *mineral oil or *tar. Although numerically unimportant, this cancer had enormous historical significance by showing that factors in the environment can cause cancer. *Benzpyrene is probably the active agent in soot and oils.

The best estimates attribute about 4% of all cancers to hazards in the workplace. Most of the occupational risks are due to *chemicals. Most cancer hazards are strictly regulated by industry and State

Table 12: Cancer-causing chemicals in industry and relative risks

Agent	Cancer	Relative Risk
Arsenic	Skin, lung	2.3–8.0
Asbestos	Lung	1.5–12.0
	Mesothelioma	100
Benzene	Leukaemia	2.5
Benzidine	Bladder	14
Bis chloro-methyl ether (BCME)	Lung	100
Coke oven emissions	Lung, kidney	2.1
Foundry gases	Lung	?
Magenta	Bladder	?
2-Naphthylamine	Bladder	87
Nickel smelting	Nasal cavities	?
Radon (uranium)	Lung	?
Vinyl chloride monomer	Liver angiosarcoma	+++
Wood dust	Nasal cavities	500

Relative risk = the number of times greater chance than the general population has of acquiring cancer. +++ = formerly a very high risk in those exposed, before the danger was recognized.

authorities. However, there is no room for complacency. New chemicals are being introduced all the time, accidents happen and regulations may be ignored. Nevertheless, the risk associated with certain

Table 13: Industrial processes and occupations associated with cancer

---

*Auramine manufacture

*Aluminium production

Boot and shoe manufacture and repair

*Chromium plating, chromium pigment

Coal gasification (older processes)

*Coke production Kidney cancers more frequent in coke oven workers

Furniture manufacture (*wood dusts)

*Iron and steel founding

Isopropyl alcohol manufacture (strong acid process)

*Magenta manufacture

*Nickel smelting and refining (nasal cavity cancer)

Radiology (*leukaemia), *medical X-rays

Rubber manufacture (leukaemia), *benzidine, *naphthylamine, *auramine, *magenta, 4-*aminobiphenyl, 4-*nitrophenyl

Underground haematite mining (exposure to *radon gas)

*Uranium mining (lung cancer)

Viticulture (*arsenic in pesticides)

*hazardous agent unknown

Table 14: Chemicals strongly suspected of being human carcinogens

Agent	Industry
acrylonitrile	plastics
beryllium and beryllium compounds	metals
creosote	wood preservation, others
diethyl sulphate	chemical
dimethyl sulphate	chemical
nickel and nickel compounds	nickel refining, welding (fumes)
ortho-toluidine	dye

chemicals in industry, particularly *asbestos, has become exaggerated in the popular imagination.

Chemicals proven to cause cancer in humans are listed in Table 13. There are undoubtedly more that have not been identified, for example in the shoe industry, in coal and coke industries and in wood dusts (Table 14). Chemicals strongly suspected of causing cancer are listed in Table 14.

A survey of workers in the petroleum industry showed a lower than average overall incidence of cancer. The cancers they did develop, however, were more commonly *leukaemias and also *lymphomas.

*Lung cancers are the most frequent cancers resulting from occupational exposure to carcinogens. It is not commonly recognised that *tobacco has had a very big influence on the emergence of industrial cancers. For example, the risk of lung cancer from *asbestos exposure, is 10 times greater among smokers than non-smokers. The same tendency is found in the *uranium and *foundry industries. In fact, most of the cancers associated with known occupational carcinogens occur in smokers.

Ochsner, Alton born 1896, Chicago surgeon, professor in Tulane, whose work was influential in confirming the association between *tobacco smoking and lung cancer

OESOPHAGUS CANCER

Cancer of the oesophagus or gullet, the food channel from mouth to stomach, is relatively infrequent in most Western countries, but very serious.

Causes of Cancer of the Oesophagus

There are many clues to the causation of oesophageal cancer. It is 300 times more common along the shores of the Caspian sea and in some areas of China than in parts of the world with the lowest incidence. Deficiency of *vitamin A and infection by a fungus (*Fusarium moniliforme*) are suspected as causes. An adequate dietary intake of *vitamin A has a protective effect against the development of oesophageal cancer. Also, people in affected areas eat a monotonous diet deficient in many nutrients, particularly the B group vitamin, *riboflavin. In South and East Africa, an epidemic was observed when maize replaced millet and sorghum as the staple food. A maize diet is deficient in many important nutrients, including *zinc and riboflavin.

In Western communities *tobacco and the heavy consumption of *alcohol are causative factors in cancer of the oesophagus. The chance of cancer of the oesophagus seems to be multiplied, rather than simply added, when both of these risks are in the equation.

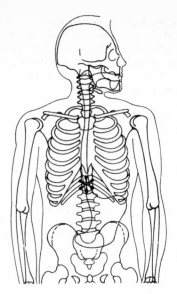

Fig. 37:
   Cancer of the oesophagus. The oesophagus (the 'gullet') is the tube leading from the mouth to the stomach. Cancer of the oesophagus is suspected when a person develops difficulty swallowing. Often the cancer is advanced when it is diagnosed, by which time it has spread into vital neighbouring structures inside the chest, so that it cannot be removed surgically.

Inflammation of the lower oesophagus, resulting from reflux of acid stomach contents, may be a causative factor. The incidence is relatively high in persons who have swallowed corrosive liquids. Persons with the uncommon condition *coeliac disease have a tendency to develop oesophageal cancer.

Symptoms of Cancer of the Oesophagus
The patient may have no symptoms until the food channel is seriously narrowed by the cancer. Difficulty in swallowing is a serious symptom that should always be investigated. X-ray examinations after the patient has swallowed a barium-containing contrast medium demonstrate most cancers, and they can also be seen through an *endoscope. The diagnosis must always be confirmed by taking a biopsy.
   Advanced oesophageal cancer may cause *pain and even starvation because of an inability to swallow. The oesophagus passes through a region containing many vital structures, including large blood vessels, the heart, major airways and nerves. Symptoms arise when these structures are invaded.

158

Treatment of Cancer of the Oesophagus

Even if the tumour is localized and and the patient receives treatment by *surgery or *radiotherapy, cancer of the oesophagus is most likely to recur. Inoperable and recurrent tumours can be treated by *chemotherapy combined with radiotherapy, but in most cases the response does not last many months.

oestrogen   class of *hormone that directs growth and development of female characteristics, such as breasts. Oestrogen is a factor in the causation of *breast and other female cancers. *Oral contraceptives contain oestrogen.

*Diethylstilboestrol, an oestrogen synthesized in the laboratory, used to be given to pregnant women in order to prevent miscarriage. Many daughters of women who received diethylstilboestrol developed cancers of the vagina at the time of puberty.

Paradoxically, oestrogens are used to treat cancer of the prostate and some cases of breast cancer. Some cells on depend on oestrogens for growth, whereas the growth of some types of cancer cells is inhibited by the same hormones.

Olympic Dam   uranium, gold, silver and copper mine near *Roxby Downs in South Australia. See *atomic bombs and nuclear reactors.

oncogene   abnormal *gene that may cause cancer. Oncogenes are faulty copies of normal genes that have been taken up by viruses and are inserted into the cells that become the hosts of the virus. The products of these faulty genes cause deregulation of growth. See *nature of cancer.

oncology   study of cancer, also practice of cancer medicine

Oncovin   trade name of medication used in cancer *chemotherapy

oral contraceptives   Oral contraceptives represent a great medical advance. They have provided a tool to combat one of humankind's greatest threats: overpopulation. By giving women a measure of control over their own lives they have been agents of great social change. They have also saved many lives by preventing dangerous pregnancies. On balance, the safety they afford outweighs their dangers.

It is estimated that 50 to 100 million women worldwide use *oral contraceptives. The oral contraceptives usually contain two female hormones, one a type of *oestrogen, or feminising hormone, and one a type of *progestin, which prepares the uterus for pregnancy. Levels of both hormones rise and fall during the 28–day female hormonal cycle. The effect of taking the hormones is to stop maturation of the ovum during the menstrual cycle and thus prevent its release from the ovary. Oral contraceptives therefore alter slightly the normal hormonal levels in women who use them.

There may be a slight increase in the risk of breast cancer in women who used combined oral contraceptives for long periods before they reached the age of 25 years. This is consistent with statistics which show that early pregnancy protects against cancer of the breast. Use over the age of 45 may also increase the risk. Combined oral contraceptives provide protection against cancer of the *uterus (endometrium) and cancer of the *ovary, while they may slightly increase the risk of cancer of the *cervix. Oestrogen alone increases the risk of endometrial cancer. See *hormonal replacement therapy.

The potential health risks to women of oral contraceptive use are not confined to cancer. Indeed, the primary risk to young women is causation of early blood vessel disease (*arteriosclerosis). For this reason, women who have high blood pressure, which also damages blood vessels, should not use the pill. The pill actually causes high blood pressure in some women. High blood cholesterol levels compound the risk of arteriosclerosis associated with oral contraceptives. These medications also increase formation of clots in veins of the leg and pelvis. Because clot formation is a risk after surgery, the pill should be stopped up to 6 weeks before a planned operation.

On balance, the risks with modern low dose contraceptives are less than than the hazards of pregnancy and abortion, and of most alternative methods of contraception. *Smoking is the overwhelming risk factor for all women on the pill, multiplying the risk of blood vessel disease: the cause of heart disease and stroke. The older the woman, the greater the risk. Women who use oral contraceptives should not smoke, and this is particularly crucial for those over 35 years of age.

Women who read reports (and they are frequent) for guidance on the use of oral contraceptives are bound to be confused, because the experts have not reached a verdict. They cannot do so, because the evidence is not all in. However, the risk of cancer accompanies all types of *oestrogen, including those a woman's body makes itself. Theoretically, oral contraceptives will not add much to the risk if they are not taken in amounts significantly greater than provided by the body itself.

organochlorines   any compound of chlorine and the organic elements carbon, hydrogen, nitrogen or oxygen. This broad class of compounds includes herbicides such as *2, 4-D, *2, 4, 5-T and *dioxin, *chlorinated insecticides and *polychlorinated biphenyls. Many organochlorines are highly toxic to living matter and some cause cancer in some species.

osteosarcoma   kind of *bone cancer

OVARY CANCER

Although cancer of the ovaries is the least common of the female genital cancers it is the most highly malignant and its incidence is increasing. In Australia approximately 1500 women develop ovarian cancer every year and until recently 75% died from their disease, usually within 2–3 years. Like other cancers it is more common in the elderly, but cancer of the ovary occurs from young adulthood on.

Cause of Ovarian Cancer

*Oestrogen is thought to be a factor. As with *breast cancer, nulliparity—failure to bear children—is a risk factor. Pregnancy is thought to reduce the effect of oestrogen.

Symptoms of Ovarian Cancer

Vague lower abdominal discomfort and backache may be the only symptoms. In advanced cancer of the ovary, the abdomen may be swollen because of the accumulation of fluid.

Diagnosis of Ovarian Cancer

Pelvic examination may reveal a tumour in the region of the ovary. Small tumours may be seen on *ultrasound imaging or *computed

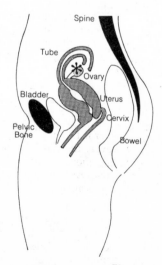

Fig. 38:

Cancer of the ovary. Ovarian cancer often causes grumbling lower abdominal discomfort which is at first thought to arise from the bowel. Expert pelvic examination and ultrasound imaging are needed to make the diagnosis.

tomography (CT) or by *laparoscopy. The diagnosis is made by biopsy during laparoscopy or *surgery, with microscopic examination of the removed tissue.

Treatment of Ovarian Cancer
*Surgery, *chemotherapy and *radiotherapy are all used to treat ovarian cancer. Major advances have been made in chemotherapy. Responses, not cures, are obtained in 80% of cases. Responses may be partial or complete. Some complete responders may relapse.

Prevention of Ovarian Cancer
Regular pelvic examination and proper investigation of lower abdominal symptoms, which are often suspected at first to arise in the bowel, may lead to earlier detection of ovarian cancer. *Ultrasound scanning is being studied for mass *screening, but screening is difficult to implement with such an expensive technique, because ovarian cancer is uncommon. As yet, there is no formal proof that early detection and treatment improve the outlook.

Oral Contraceptives and Ovarian Cancer
Three studies have now shown a significant reduction of risk of ovarian cancer in women who have used *oral contraceptives. The protection against ovarian cancer is thought to last 15 or more years after use of the pill has stopped. Since there are risks from the contraceptive pill, including clot formation, high blood pressure and a possible increase in risk from *breast cancer, the pill cannot be recommended as a prophylactic against ovarian cancer.

ozone layer   layer of a form of oxygen (O_3) high in the upper atmosphere (the stratosphere, above 10km), which reduces the intensity of *ultraviolet light reaching the Earth's surface. The ozone layer has been reduced by the accumulation of fluorohydrocarbons used as refrigerants and as propellants in spray cans. It has been estimated that deterioration of the ozone layer will result in a 50% increase of *skin cancer over the next 20 years. In the past few years, the rate of skin cancer has gone up exactly as would be expected from the corresponding loss of ozone.

The concentration of ozone in the lower atmosphere (the troposphere, below 10 km) is actually increasing in the northern hemisphere and this may counteract the reduction in the stratosphere. Measurements in Bavaria actually showed a decrease, from 1968 to 1982, in UVB, the carcinogenic fraction of ultraviolet light, reaching the Earth's surface at noon.

Ozone is formed by the interaction of hydrocarbons with *nitrogen oxides.

P

Paget, Sir James 1814–1899, celebrated English surgeon who became professor of surgery at the Royal College of Surgeons in 1847 and was elected a Fellow of the Royal Society in 1851. Besides the diseases of bone and the nipple named after him, he was the first to describe two other diseases and wrote books on surgery, tumours and other diseases. His private practice made him very wealthy and he became surgeon to the Queen.

Paget's disease of bone non-malignant disease causing thickening of bone, in which *bone cancer sometimes occurs

Paget's disease of the breast type of *breast cancer usually spreading from deeper in the breast to involve the nipple

pain In the healthy body, pain is a warning signal. Cancer is often entirely painless, but sometimes it causes the most severe pain.

The perception of pain depends on many factors. Pain is only perceived by the sufferer. The doctor must interpret what he is told by the patient. The experienced doctor knows that fear, depression and anxiety intensify pain. It is common knowledge that soldiers in war may suffer awful injuries, but only become aware of them after the battle. Then they experience pain.

The commonest reason for pain in cancer is its spread to bones. If the bones of the spine are invaded by cancer, they frequently fracture, causing pressure on nerves. Another cause of pain is involvement of the lining of the lungs, giving rise to *pleurisy, a pain in the chest made worse by breathing.

Pain in patients with cancer is commonly not caused by the cancer, but by another illness or complication. Patients with cancer may, of course, also suffer problems that beset non-cancer patients. It is the job of the doctor to make a correct diagnosis of the cause of pain in every instance.

Treatment of pain depends on the cause. If the pain is due to cancer, the best way to treat it is to bring about a retreat of the cancer, if that is possible. This may be effected by *surgery, *radiotherapy or *chemotherapy, according to the circumstances.

Pain-relieving medications will control all pains, if prescribed properly and used correctly. Simple non-narcotic analgesic agents like aspirin and paracetamol control many pains. More severe pain requires narcotic medications which are all related to morphine. Often the requirement for narcotic agents can be reduced by judicious use of simple pain-relievers, anti-rheumatic medications, anti-emetics, anti-depressants and medications of the *cortisone class. Too often patients are reluctant to take strong pain-relieving medications, through fear of *addiction, or in the mistaken notion that the medication will not be effective when it is really needed.

Even today, patients are denied sufficient pain relief because of old-fashioned attitudes by medical and nursing staff. The patient in hospital has a right to have his or her pain prescription discussed by the doctor in the presence of the nurse in charge, so that there can be no doubt what measures are to be taken if pain occurs. A prescription for pain relief is a very individual matter. Doses required for adequate relief of pain very widely and the perception of pain is highly individual. Only the patient really knows how much medication he or she needs.

In 1680, Thomas *Sydenham, celebrated English physician, wrote: 'Among the remedies which it has pleased Almighty God to give man to relieve his sufferings, none is so universal and so efficacious as opium'. The same is true today.

Addiction to narcotic medications is rarely a serious problem in patients with cancer. The requirement of most patients for narcotics stops when an operation or radiotherapy relieves the pain. In the case of many cancer patients who would otherwise suffer pain, dependence on narcotic agents is no disaster when the alternatives are considered.

When pain is a severe problem, medication should be taken regularly, each dose acting to prevent the return of pain.

Newer approaches to pain include spinal injections, instruments that deliver slow pain-relieving infusions and cutaneous electrical counter-stimulation. Cancer centres usually have pain clinics to which patients with resistant pain may be referred.

*Morphine may be injected directly into the fluid around the spine to gain control of pain when there is no response to morphine given by injection or by mouth.

The best way of controlling bone pain due to cancer is to cause the tumour to regress by radiotherapy, or appropriate chemotherapy with cytotoxic drugs or hormones. Bone pain often responds to radiotherapy, but radiotherapy cannot be given twice to the same site. A new approach is to use *radioactive chemicals that home in on bone tumours. One such chemical under study is samarium-153, which has a very short lifetime, so that the patient is not exposed to unnecessary irradiation.

PANCREAS CANCER

The pancreas is in the back of the abdomen, extending from the midline across to the left. It makes juices which pass into the small bowel to digest the food. It is also the site of glands which make insulin.

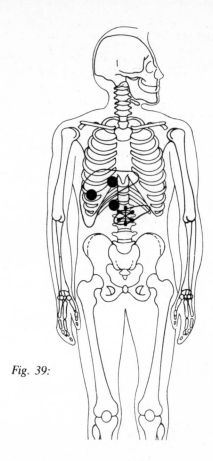

Fig. 39:

Cancer of the pancreas. The pancreas, which makes digestive juices, lies at the back of the abdomen. Tumours developing in this gland do not at first cause abnormal sensations. A tumour may block the bile duct, causing jaundice. Prostatic cancer often spreads to the liver.

Cause of Pancreatic Cancer

We do not know all of the factors causing carcinoma of the pancreas. *Tobacco is a contributory factor and *diet is suspected. Coffee has been questioned, but no firm evidence has been obtained to incriminate it.

Symptoms of Pancreatic Cancer

Cancer of the pancreas often causes no symptoms early in its development. It frequently comes to notice when it has blocked the bile duct, causing *jaundice. The patient may lose weight or have pain in the back.

Diagnosis of Pancreatic Cancer

Pancreatic cancers are difficult to diagnose because the pancreas is hard to see on X-rays, *CT scans and *ultrasound pictures. Sometimes the disease can be diagnosed by obtaining tissue using an *endoscope passed through the stomach and upper small intestine into the pancreatic duct. Often the cancer is diagnosed by obtaining a *biopsy during surgery.

Treatment of Pancreatic Cancer

Cancer of the pancreas is rarely curable, and responds poorly to treatment.

*Pain can be a very serious problem with this cancer, requiring specialist help. Pain nerves can be injected in the spine or cut, and other special measures may be needed to deliver pain-relieving medications into the spinal canal or to ensure a constant supply of drug to the body.

Fortunately, the incidence of cancer of the pancreas has been declining in the past 10 years.

Papanicolaou, George 1883–1962, a Greek-born American anatomist, Professor at Cornell University, New York. His studies led to the development of Papanicolaou staining ('Pap' stain), for *smear tests of the cervix, to detect abnormal or cancer cells. See *cervix cancer.

papilloma virus family of viruses causing warts in animals and humans. Particular types of human papilloma viruses are causative agents of *cervix cancer.

Pap smear see *Papanicolaou and *smear test

parotid glands tissues below the ears and behind the jaws that make saliva, which become enlarged in mumps, sometimes the site of tumours which may be *benign or *malignant. *Surgery presents the difficulty of removing the gland without damaging the nerve to the muscles of the face, which passes through the parotid gland. Damage to the facial nerve leads to paralysis of the facial muscles on that side.

passive smoking inhalation of smoke from other persons' *tobacco smoke. Many studies have confirmed the first report from Japan in 1981 that passive smoking increases the risk of *lung cancer. The Japanese studied 92,000 non-smoking women, of whom about one in four were married to smokers. The women were followed up for 14 years, by which time 174 had died of lung cancer. The mortality rate in non-smokers married to smokers was 60% higher than in non-smokers married to non-smokers, after eliminating factors of age and occupation.

It has been estimated that 17–25% of lung cancer deaths in non-smokers may be attributed to passive smoking. According to information from the UK passive smoking causes 100–200 deaths a year in non-smokers.

The smoke that the smoker draws into his lungs is called **mainstream smoke** and the smoke given off by a cigarette between puffs is called **sidestream smoke.** In sidestream smoke there is about three times the amount of *benzepyrene as there is in mainstream smoke. The amount of benzepyrene that is taken in by a single non-smoker, among several smokers, in an unventilated office, can be as much as the smokers inhale. Sidestream smoke also contains about 50 times more *nitrosamines than does mainstream smoke.

pathology   study of disease processes as they affect *tissues. Knowledge of pathology is applied to microscopic diagnosis of diseases in tissues obtained by *biopsy.

penis cancer   Cancer of the penis is uncommon in Western countries, representing less than 0.1% of all male cancers, but it is fairly common in many developing countries in Central and South America, Africa, and in some provinces in China, wherever *circumcision is not practised and poor hygiene abounds. The highest incidence of cancer of the penis is in Uganda and Brazil, where relatively young men, aged 33–35 years, are affected. *Papilloma virus has been implicated in cases which have been tested, but other factors, including foreskin secretions and inflammation are considered to be contributory factors.

Around the world, the incidence of cancer of the penis is related to whether or not circumcision is carried out. Cancer of the penis is most frequent in the uncircumcised.

pernicious anaemia   disease characterized by *anaemia resulting from degeneration of the stomach, leading to a failure to to absorb *vitamin B12. Persons who have pernicious anaemia have a greater risk of *stomach cancer.

pesticide   see *chlorinated insecticides, *air pollution

Peters, M. Vera   Canadian radiotherapist who showed, in a series of studies from 1950 on, that *Hodgkin's disease could be cured by adequate radiotherapy.

P-Glycoprotein

P-glycoprotein substance building up in tumour cells in response to *chemotherapy, enabling them to pump out the chemotherapeutic medication, thereby conferring resistance to this form of treatment

phenacetin analgesic drug which, if abused, may cause cancers of the *bladder and *ureter

photodynamic therapy cancer treatment which allows tumour cells to be attacked in a way somewhat different from all other methods of treatment. Some light-sensitive substances will localize in tumours after they have been injected into the bloodstream. A light directed at the sensitized tumour, usually through a light-conducting fibre connected to a *laser, activates the chemical, which then kills cells in its vicinity.

placebo treatment, which has no active ingredient, given to humour a patient. The 'placebo effect' is easily demonstrated with mildly to moderately severe pain. If, in a *clinical trial a group of patients given a tablet, for example, is compared with a group given no tablet, there is usually some pain relief from the tablet, even though it contains only an absolutely inactive substance.

The placebo effect is greater when the placebo is given with suggestion and reassurance. When a new treatment comes along, as happens frequently, the first trials are reported enthusiastically and optimistically. See *alternative cancer treatments, clinical trials.

placenta the afterbirth, an organ that develops in pregnancy and enables the developing baby to obtain nourishment from the mother. The baby is attached to the placenta by the umbilical cord. Cancer of the placenta, called choriocarcinoma, is uncommon. Choriocarcinoma may arise during a pregnancy that produces only a grossly abnormal placenta, called a hydatidiform mole, or it may follow miscarriages, abnormal or normal pregnancies. Treatment with *chemotherapy is sometimes necessary and is frequently curative.

platelets small blood cells lacking nuclei (as do red cells), which control bleeding by plugging small holes in blood vessels and by starting the clotting reaction when vessels are cut. Patients deficient in platelets have a tendency to bleed spontaneously or after minor injury. See *chemotherapy.

pleura membrane covering the lungs and lining the inside of the chest

pleurisy particular type of *pain, arising in *pleura. Pleurisy is usually a sharp or stabbing pain in the chest, made worse by breathing or coughing

pollution   see *air pollution, *water

polonium-210   highly radioactive metal, discovered in the mineral pitchblend by Marie *Curie in 1898. It also occurs in *uranium ores and, in trace amounts, in *tobacco smoke. Polonium-210 has a half-life of 138.4 days. Polonium is produced in nuclear reactors and by atomic bombs. See *metals.

polychlorinated biphenyls (PCB)   chemicals once widely used in electrical equipment, suspected of playing a part in causing *malignant melanoma, listed by the US Environmental Protection Agency as carcinogens. PCBs also have other biological effects in animals, including infertility and miscarriage. Production in the USA was stopped in 1977 following passage of the Toxic Substances Control Act, but PCBs are very stable and persist in the environment. Huge quantities (270 million kg) have been dumped on land and sea. Traces of PCBs have been found in virtually every living species and in every stretch of land and water examined. Australian PCB waste is disposed of by shipping it to Wales in the UK, where it is incinerated. PCB can be degraded by a microorganism called white rot fungus and by particular species of non-toxic bacteria. It is hoped that it will be economical to set up commercial plants that will deal with PCB waste at the rate of tens of tonnes per week.

POLYCYCLIC HYDROCARBONS
The polycyclic hydrocarbons are based on multiples of *benzene, a compound of carbon and hydrogen with a molecular structure in the form of a hexagon. Benzene itself is an important constituent of

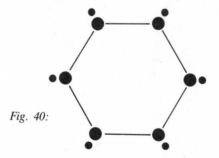

Fig. 40:

Benzene. Benzene is a component of motor fuels and a very common constituent of living matter. Many compounds containing several benzene rings (polycyclic hydrocarbons) are carcinogenic. It is a six-sided chemical compound made up of carbon (large) and hydrogen (small) atoms.

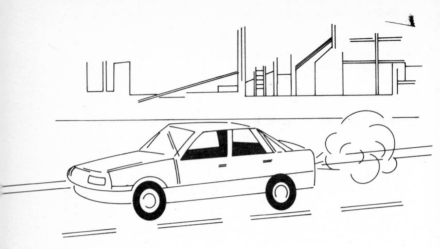

Fig. 41:

Benzepyrene is funnelled into the atmosphere. Benzepyrene is a polycyclic hydrocarbon *chemical substance that is inevitably formed when oils, animal and vegetable matter are burned. Benzepyrene causes cancer in experimental animals and is undoubtedly a factor in the causation of human cancers, particularly as an environmental pollutant.*

*tobacco smoke. Polycyclic hydrocarbons are everywhere in the environment. They are distilled from coal *tar and they also arise in cooking. A member of this family of substances, *dimethyl-benzanthracene (DMBA) can cause cancer of the skin, lung, stomach and ovaries, as well as leukaemia, in experimental animals. The kind of tumour which develops depends both on the animal and on how the carcinogen is administered.

*Benzepyrene, a polycyclic hydrocarbon compound proven to be a carcinogen and universally accepted as such, is found in the air of large cities in concentrations as high as 400 micrograms per thousand cubic metres. It is constantly funnelled into the atmosphere from chimneys and exhaust pipes. Cooking fats and oils may contain up to 20 micrograms per kilogram, vegetables up to 25, and the concentration on the outside of a charcoal-grilled steak may reach 50 micrograms per kilogram. Humans have been eating benzepyrene since they began cooking food.

It has been clearly shown that benzepyrene is bound to the *DNA of a large proportion of normal subjects who live in big cities. In animals treated with this compound, the number of cancers that

170

develop increases in proportion to the amount of benzepyrene that binds to DNA.

polyp branching growth that protrudes from the wall of the bowel, bladder or other *epithelium

potassium-40 weakly radioactive form of potassium that is mixed with all forms of potassium and therefore taken up in the body, constituting 1 gram of the 100 grams in the body. Potassium-40 is one source of the unavoidable or background *radiation to which we are all exposed.

Pott, Percivall b 1714, London surgeon who recognized the association of soot with *scrotum cancer in chimney sweeps. He worked at St. Bartholomew's Hospital and wrote many other important papers on surgery, the first of which described the type of fracture of the leg, now known as Pott's fracture, which he sustained when thrown from a horse.

power lines A link has been suggested recently between radio waves and cancer. Radio waves are a form of *electromagnetic radiation. Above average numbers of cancers have been reported in ham radio operators, as has an unusually high incidences of leukaemia among children who live near power lines. This evidence is weak and inconsistent. One problem with *epidemiological studies of cancer is the difficulty in accounting for other factors. For example, accommodation near power lines may be relatively cheap, attracting underprivileged people whose diet may be lacking essential nutrients or may contain carcinogens. There is a higher incidence of cancer among people in lower *socioeconomic classes.

A study of 147,000 cases over a 20–year period, using the Swedish cancer environment register, suggested an increased risk of chronic lymphocytic *leukaemia for electronic and electrical power engineers and technicians. In a recent review of eleven studies the risk of electrical workers for acute myeloid leukaemia was found to be 1.46 times the normal risk.

The question of the risk of magnetic fields also arises in the case of *'maglev' trains. Some home appliances, such as electric blankets also expose users to magnetic fields.

Magnetic fields are measured in units called 'tesla'. The greatest strength of the Earth's magnetic field reaches 67 microtesla (thousandths of a tesla). The largest power lines generate magnetic fields of about 40 tesla.

prednisolone, prednisone cortisone-type hormonal medications, frequently used in cancer *chemotherapy

pregnancy and X-rays see *X-rays

PREVENTION OF CANCER
Primary prevention is removal or avoidance of the factors which cause cancer. As individuals we may not be able to change the hazards in the world around us, but we can institute sensible rules of living that offer us the best chance of avoiding cancer. The largest cancer risk factors are the ones we can control, and of these *diet and *tobacco are by far the biggest.

There are still many unknowns in cancer, but if we used what we know already, the incidence of cancer could be reduced substantially. Some guidelines are stated here.

General Guidelines for Reducing Cancer Risks—Primary Prevention of Cancer
1. Do not smoke and avoid exposure to *tobacco smoke (*passive smoking).
2. Avoid *obesity.
3. Increase consumption of foods containing *vitamins A, C, D and *E.
4. Ensure an adequate intake of minerals, particularly zinc and selenium. (3) and (4) are best achieved by having a varied and mixed *diet. See *mineral deficiency and cancer.
5. Reduce consumption of animal *fats.
6. Regulate intake of *alcohol. There are many reasons why alcohol consumption should not exceed an average of two drinks a day. At least one day per week should be alcohol-free.
7. Avoid sexually-transmitted viruses. See *papilloma virus, *AIDS.
8. If possible do not take medications and *hormones known to be carcinogenic. See *oral contraceptives, *hormone replacement therapy, *chemotherapy, *medical treatment as a cause of cancer.
9. Be alert to the possibility of environmental contamination. Avoid using carcinogenic chemicals. See *chemicals as causes of cancer, *air pollution, *water.
10. Avoid excessive exposure to sunlight and use *sunscreens. See *ultraviolet light.
11. Have medical examination when you perceive a *warning sign.
12. Have appropriate *screening tests. See *mammography, *cervix cancer, *prostate cancer.

The big question is what is the cost:benefit ratio for each of our environmental and lifestyle hazards? How many lives would be gained by eliminating them, and at what cost? Are there substitutes? The cost of removing asbestos from old buildings is enormous. For that cost, could more lives have been saved in other ways? These are the questions which have to be faced if we are to make the best terms with the cancer problem and governments must make many of the decisions about the use of carcinogens. However, most of the choices affecting the development of cancer must be taken by the individual.

Secondary Prevention—Early Diagnosis of Cancer

Secondary prevention of cancer is the cure of early cancers. Cancer of the cervix is a good example. An early cervical cancer is a small patch of malignant cells, not more than a few cells deep. Removal of this patch is completely effective in curing the cancer. Cancer can be diagnosed earlier in the community by combining better public education with *screening tests. See also *breast, *prostate, *large bowel and *cervix cancers.

New tissue stains to enable the pathologist to distinguish early cancers from benign conditions. Some of these stains use monoclonal *antibodies. *Computed tomography (CT) *ultrasound imaging, *mammography and *magnetic resonance imaging (MRI), can now provide us with pictures of bodily organs of previously unimagined clarity, permitting earlier diagnosis of cancer.

It would be better if active preventive measures could be taken by women with a family history of *breast cancer, rather than relying on constant observation. Because women's own female hormones (*oestrogens) are involved in the development of breast cancer, drugs that block the effect of oestrogen are being considered. *Tamoxifen, the best drug available for this purpose, is effective in the treatment of a proportion of cases of incurable breast cancer, but proper trials have not yet been carried out. However, the side effects of tamoxifen should not be overlooked. See *tamoxifen, *chemoprevention.

*Adjuvant chemotherapy for women who have had a breast cancer operation—*mastectomy or *lumpectomy—in whom no cancer cells have been found in the lymph nodes removed at the time of the operation, is a difficult issue. About 30% of these patients, untreated, will have relapse within 4 years. See *breast cancer.

Procarbazine   medication used in cancer *chemotherapy

progestin   class of female hormones, also known as progestagen, made by the ovary in the second part of the menstrual cycle, essential for the fertilized ovum to be retained and develop in the uterus. The most important natural progestin is *progesterone. Progestins tend to raise the level of some classes of fat in the blood, increasing the risk of *arteriosclerosis or blood vessel damage. See *oral contraceptive, *breast and *kidney cancer.

primary cancer   designation of the original tumour, as distinct from *secondary or *metastatic tumour.

progesterone   female hormone of the *progestin class.

Promoter

promoter agent that fosters development of cancer in tissues that have been exposed to an *initiator. Cancer usually results from exposure to more than one agent. After exposure to an initiator, further exposure to a *promoter is required for the full development of a cancer. On their own, cancer promoters do not cause cancer. See *initiator, *causation of cancer.

PROSTATE CANCER
In males the prostate gland surrounds the urethra, the tube leading from the bladder. The gland, which makes the seminal fluid, almost always enlarges in later life in response to hormonal stimuli. Mostly the enlargement is due to benign tissue.

Prostatic cancer is the commonest tumour of elderly men in developed Western countries. In post-mortem examinations microscopic foci of prostatic cancer are found in more than 80% of old men. These foci grow very slowly in most old men, causing no trouble. The incidence of prostatic cancer has risen quite steeply in black American men so that they have 50% more prostatic cancer than white men in USA.

Cause of Cancer of the Prostate
The cause of prostate cancer is not known. Men who have smoked for many years have a two to threefold risk of prostatic cancer. Vasectomy and early age of first intercourse are suggested minor risk factors that have not been proven.

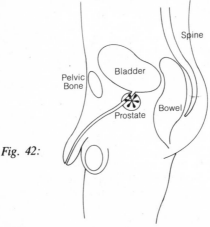

Fig. 42:

Cancer of the prostate. The male prostate gland surrounds the urethra, the tube leading from the bladder. It makes seminal fluid. Both benign enlargement and cancer cause the outlet from the bladder to become narrowed or obstructed.

Symptoms of Cancer of the Prostate

Unfortunately, the cancer may cause no symptoms until it is advanced. Enlargement of the gland, affecting most elderly men, whether benign or malignant, causes symptoms of slow flow of urine and frequent desire to empty the bladder.

Prostatic cancer may be detected on routine examination in men over 50 years of age. The physician can feel the posterior surface of the gland with a gloved finger in the rectum. Sometimes cancer is

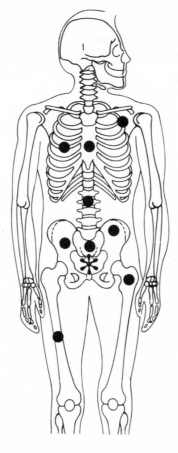

Fig. 43:

Spread of prostate cancer. Prostate cancer has a particular tendency to spread to bones. It also spreads locally and to other sites.

discovered at operation through the urethra—transurethral resection—to open up the urethra narrowed by growth of the prostate. Nonmalignant growth of the prostate gland is common in elderly men, with narrowing of the urethra. Advanced prostatic cancer spreads into bones, often causing *pain.

Diagnosis of Cancer of the Prostate
The essential biopsy for microscopic proof of cancer can, in many cases, be obtained under local anaesthetic through a hollow needle. Otherwise it is obtained during surgery. Sometimes the X-ray appearances of advanced prostatic cancer in bones are typical and high levels of a compound produced by prostatic cancer cells (acid phosphatase) may be found in the blood.

Treatment of Cancer of the Prostate
There are a number of unanswered questions in the treatment of prostatic cancer, which is the reason why experts differ. Early prostatic cancer is often cured by surgical removal of most of the gland. Tumours that have spread to the surface of the gland and beyond can usually be treated successfully by *radiotherapy.

Patients are often concerned that operation on the prostate will cause loss of sexual potency. Loss of erections rarely follows transurethral resection, but may be a problem after bigger operations.

The growth of prostatic cancer is often inhibited by treatment with *oestrogen or newer drugs, or by removing the supply of male hormone, which entails removal of the testes. Whether to use oestrogen or to castrate the patient early in the course of the disease is an unsolved controversy, because it has not been proved that either of these measures will improve survival. They are instigated in the hope of retarding the spread of the cancer to bones and thus reducing the symptoms associated with this.

When the tumour is no longer controlled by hormonal measures, the pain of prostatic cancer in bones may respond to *radiotherapy.

Prevention of Cancer of the Prostate
Men over the age of 50 should have a rectal examination yearly. This is a cheap and effective *screening test.

protein major class of body substances (other major classes are *carbohydrates and *fats). All cells contain many kinds of protein. Some proteins are *enzymes, others have a structural function. Movement of cells, for example contraction of muscle cells, depends on special types of protein.

A protein is made by stringing together the basic building blocks, *amino acids. The nature and function of proteins depend on the sequence and number of *amino acids in the chain. The order in

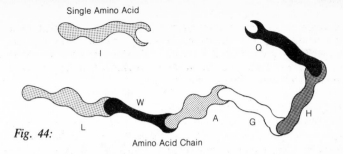

Single Amino Acid

Fig. 44:

Amino Acid Chain

The nature of protein. Proteins are simply long strings of chemical units called amino acids. After they are joined head to tail, they take up their own shape. There are 20 amino acids that are used throughout nature. Proteins may be long cables, flat sheets, tangled skeins or tubular structures. All these shapes are determined primarily by the sequence of the amino acids, because some form an angle with their neighbours, some are attracted to other amino acids in the chain and others repel each other. Nature achieves infinite variety through the combinations of the 20 amino acids. There is a one-letter shorthand code for the names of the amino acids. I = isoleucine, L = leucine, W = tryptophane etc.

which the amino acids are joined together is specified by the *genes for each protein, according to the rules of the *genetic code.

The shape of a protein is determined by the way each amino acid accommodates to its neighbours. Some amino acids repel each other, others are attracted to each other. As a result, the most complex shapes can result. Protein can form long threads, tangles and sheets. The shape of proteins is modified by their chemical environment. By changing their environment, proteins can be made to work, pushing, pulling, grasping substances and bringing materials together so that they can be joined.

The production of protein is described under *nature of cancer.

pyelogram X-ray examination of the kidneys, ureters and bladder. The X-ray image is obtained after intravenous injection of a contrast medium that is concentrated and excreted by the kidneys.

R

radiation In the 16th century the miners of the Schneeberg-Jachimov region of Bohemia developed a fatal lung disease, which was eventually shown to be *lung cancer. The cause of the disease is now known to have been radioactivity in the mines. It is now recognised that radiation, in the form of short wavelength *electromagnetic radiation (for example *X-rays and gamma rays) or as beams of atomic particles from *radioactive chemicals, causes cancer. The higher the dose, the greater the likelihood of cancer. Radiation causes cancer by damaging *DNA.

In modern times, lung cancers have been recorded in underground workers in uranium, fluorspar and zinc mines, resulting from inhalation of the *radon gas emanating from *radium present in the ores. The average period between exposure and the development of cancers is 20 years and *tobacco smoking substantially increases the risk.

In addition to these kinds of radiation, *ultraviolet light causes skin cancers.

There is a cancer risk with all doses of X-rays, no matter how small, and the risk is cumulative (that is, it adds up from year to year). Mankind has always been exposed to low levels of natural irradiation, from *cosmic rays from space and from natural radioactive substances. We are unavoidably exposed to radon and to weakly radioactive *potassium-40, which amounts to 1 gram of the 100 or more grams of potassium in the body. It is not possible to avoid these hazards in our life on this planet, but the risk from background irradiation appears to be very small. It has been estimated that background radiation causes 1.6% of all fatal cancers in the UK. Substantially higher doses of radiation are necessary to increase cancer risks significantly and radiation has become a serious hazard only in recent times.

High energy X-rays that can produce cancer come from *radioactive chemicals, *nuclear reactors and uranium mines. See *medical treatment as a cause of cancer.

Radioactive materials, including *radium-226 and *radium-228 were used as a paint for luminous watch dials in the 1920s. Of 2000 American women employed in the industry, using radioactive paints, 62 developed bone cancer (*osteosarcoma) and 32 developed cancers of the nasal cavities. At the most, one case of cancer of these types would normally have been expected in 2000 women.

*Radium-224 was given to children with bone tuberculosis at a private clinic in Germany shortly before World War II. A young paediatrician, *Heinz Spiess, spoke out against the practice and secured the records of the patients despite the opposition of the director of the clinic. As radium-224 has a short half life (only 3.5 days), the radioactivity affected the patients over a few months, at most. Spiess documented that radium-224 produced cancers of bone 5 to 10 years later.

As late as 1950, a preparation called *Thorotrast was used in X-ray examination of blood vessels. Thorotrast contained *thorium-223, a radioactive element which has an extremely long half-life. Thorotrast caused a very large number of deaths from cancers of the *liver and other organs. The average time between the administration of Thorotrast and development of liver cancer is 19 years.

X-rays and radioactive substances are not absolutely safe at any dose. The likelihood of cancer resulting from X-rays is proportional to the dose and this corresponds to the likelihood and extent of damage to *DNA. Within limits, damage to DNA can be repaired, but if the repair is not accurate, a *mutation results.

The adult tissues most susceptible to the carcinogenic effect of X-irradiation are those which are growing or replacing old cells most frequently—skin, lining of stomach and bowel, and blood-forming tissues in the *bone marrow. Tissues that have to replace lost cells rarely (e.g. the liver and the connective tissues) are relatively insensitive to the carcinogenic effects of X-irradiation.

radioactive chemicals substances containing elements that break down spontaneously and emit *electromagnetic radiations or subatomic particles. See *radiation, *medical treatment as a cause of cancer.

radioiodine a radioactive form of iodine, used in the treatment of overactivity of the thyroid gland and of *thyroid cancer. When used in this way, radioiodine does not cause cancer. See *iodine-131.

RADIOTHERAPY
Radiotherapy is treatment with beams of X-rays and other types of rays from radioactive sources. Radiation used to treat cancer may be generated electrically, in a linear accelerator, or come from *radioactive chemicals such as radioactive cobalt. Another source, *radium, can be placed in or close to the cancer in the form of implants or seeds, permitting a high radiation dose to be given with little damage to the nearby normal tissue. Most commonly, the radiation is beamed from an X-ray-generating machine. X-rays used in treatment are similar to those used for taking diagnostic pictures, but the dose is higher. As with X-rays used for diagnosis, the much more powerful treatment rays cannot be seen or felt passing through the body.

No form of radiation therapy makes the patient radioactive permanently and there is no radiation risk to family members or other persons.

Radiotherapy can be given with the intention of curing the patient, or of controlling symptoms. Radiotherapy to a tumour will fail to cure the cancer if cancer cells have already spread to other parts of the

179

body. Types of cancer which may be cured by radiation treatment include *head and neck (larynx, tongue), *cervix, *oesophagus and *testis cancers, *Hodgkin's disease and others.

Radiotherapy depends on cancer tissue being more sensitive than normal tissues to the damaging effects of X-rays. It is not possible to attempt cure by radiotherapy if the dose of X-rays sufficient to kill the tumour also kills too much normal tissue. Once the limit of X-ray dosage has been given, radiotherapy cannot be repeated to the same region of the body, at any later time in the life of the patient, because any more rays would cause irreparable damage to the normal tissues. Unless every cancer cell is killed, the tumour will regrow. Radiotherapy often resembles *chemotherapy, in that the more sensitive cells die, leaving the more resistant cells as sources of new and more resistant tumours.

Some tumours are regularly sensitive to X-rays, while other are insensitive. An example of a cancer sensitive to X-rays is *breast cancer.

Some tumours respond to treatment with X-rays, but are not cured by it. This is the case with most cases of *lung cancer. It is possible, in fact, to cure a proportion of very early lung cancers by radiotherapy, but in most cases treatment with X-rays does not increase the lifespan of patients with this disease. Neither radiotherapy nor *surgery can cure if the cancer has already spread outside the field of treatment. Recurrences are usually due to the presence of small secondary tumours which are undetectable at the time of the primary treatment.

Side Effects of Radiotherapy

Some patients have no troublesome side effects at all from radiotherapy. Others experience *nausea and skin reactions. Nausea is not usually a problem unless large volumes of the body are being treated near the stomach. It can generally be controlled satisfactorily by appropriate medications, but patients often lose their appetites for a while. The skin reactions are like sunburn. They are usually controlled by creams. Depending on dosage and treatment site, radiation may also cause loss of hair, cough, dry mouth or diarrhoea.

It is important to protect the area being treated from rubbing or tight clothing, and to avoid hot or cold applications to the skin. Only prescribed skin medications and lotions should be applied.

Radiation can be a particularly good way of dealing with *pain, bleeding or pressure from tumours. Treatment for painful cancer deposits in bone often requires only a short course and causes few side effects. Treatment that is intended to cure is usually given in daily doses over several weeks.

Today radiotherapy is a very sophisticated science. Treatment is individualised for each patient, often by computer matching of his or her X-ray pictures with the delivery by X-ray machines. Different types of rays are used for different sites and tumours.

Since the machines cost hundreds of thousands of dollars, radiotherapy is usually carried out in large centres. The need to travel to such a centre is one disadvantage of radiotherapy.

radium   radioactive element usually isolated by processing of uranium ores. Radium is derived from the breakdown of *uranium. It exists in several forms, all radioactive, in the natural breakdown series from uranium-238. The longest lived form, radium-226, with a *half-life of 1,622 years, was first isolated by Pierre and Marie *Curie from the ore called pitchblend. Half-lives of radium-224 and radium-228 are 3.6 days and 6.7 years respectively. See *radiation.

radon   an invisible, odourless and tasteless radioactive gas that is naturally present in the air in very low concentrations. As uranium decays, radium is formed, then the radium breaks down to radon. Radon seeps from the ground into the atmosphere. Air is drawn from the soil under a house and radon is concentrated in houses by the suction caused by chimneys, fires, fans and wind blowing around the house. In cold weather the air in a house may be replaced by outside air every two hours, resulting in great loss of heat. In cold climates measures to reduce this energy loss result in greater concentrations of radon indoors.

When radon was found trapped under houses in the United States newspaper headlines described the gas as 'a silent killer all around us'. No house in the USA escapes infiltration by radon. Its concentration depends upon the types of soil and rock underlying the house and the rate of ventilation of the house. The average dose of radiation from radon in the USA is about 3 times larger than the dose most people get from X-rays and other medical procedures in a lifetime. Americans at the higher end of the scale (hundreds of thousands of people) receive a yearly dose of radiation from their houses equal to that received by people living near *Chernobyl in 1986.

Since there is a risk of inducing cancer from irradiation, no matter how small the dose, and since the exposure to radon is life-long, radon has to be accepted as a cause of cancers. These are mainly of the *lung, because it is breathed in. The radon risk has been taken seriously by many Americans. The US Environmental Protection Agency has calculated that radon is responsible for between 5000 and 20,000 deaths per year in the USA. The risk appears to be far greater for smokers than for nonsmokers. Radon detectors are available in hardware stores in the USA.

One way of looking at the risk is to consider that if radon causes 13,000 deaths per year in USA, 11,000 of them are in smokers. Put another way, although radon causes cancers, far fewer would die if they did not smoke. The best defence against radon-induced lung cancer is to avoid *tobacco smoke and, in temperate climates, to leave windows open.

Many US cities are built on a granite base, which produces far more radon gas than, for example, Sydney's sandstone base. The levels in Britain are nearly as high as the average in America, and are higher in the south-west. One estimate suggests that a proportion (20-25%) of cases of one type of acute *leukaemia (acute myeloid) in the UK are due to natural indoor radon exposure. It is believed that the only areas in Australia where radon build-up could be a problem are near uranium deposits in the Northern Territory, but even here, good ventilation alone probably deals with the hazard. Measurements of radon in various parts of Australia have shown that there is no problem. Figures suggest that about 0.5% of lung cancer in Melbourne may be caused by exposure to radon, and those cases occur in smokers. See *tobacco.

The radon burden can be reduced greatly by appropriate measures. Sealing the floors is not very effective. In the USA the commonest practice is to drill through the basement floor to the crushed stone ballast below and to pump the air continuously from this region out of the house.

It seems inevitable that the radon risk will be taken seriously outside of the USA. Those interested may find authoritative information in two papers: 'Indoor radon: the deadliest pollutant' by Richard A Kerr, Science volume 240, page 606, (1980), and 'Controlling indoor pollution' by AV Nero, Scientific American, volume 258, page 42 (May 1988).

Ramazzani, Bernardino   1633–1714, professor of medicine in Modena and Padua, who recognized that cancer of the *cervix occurred rarely in nuns. He published a text 'De morbis artificum diatriba' that became the starting point, probably for a century, for all subsequent books on diseases of tissues. He also published early studies on the epidemiology of various diseases.

receptor   *protein structure in cells to which *growth factors and *hormones blind. The binding reaction initiates a chain of biochemical processes necessary for *growth. See *nature of cancer.

recombinant gene technology   *see genetic engineering

rectum   lower end of the large bowel. See *bowel cancer.

remission   disappearance of detectable cancer resulting spontaneously or from treatment. The term 'remission' is used in distinction from *cure, which is often defined as remission lasting 5 or 10 years.

retinoblastoma   an uncommon malignant tumour that develops at the back of the eye in children. In the majority of cases the condition is inherited, due to an abnormality of a *chromosome (*see heredity and cancer). Retinoblastoma also occurs sporadically, in subjects with no family history of the disease.

Retinoblastoma is treatable when caught early, but survivors have a higher than normal risk of developing other cancers later in life, particularly *osteosarcoma. The curative treatment is *surgery, to remove the affected eye.

retinoic acid   *retinoid compound. See *alternative cancer treatments.

retinoids   substances of the *vitamin A family that appear to inhibit the development and growth of some cancers. Retinoid compounds, currently used in the treatment of acne, are being tested for their capacity to prevent *skin cancer and ageing of skin. Retinoids accumulate primarily in the skin. They are thought to act by enhancing the normal *differentiation and *growth of *epithelium of skin and other tissues. Retinoids protect against *mutations in experimental animals caused by various chemicals. Two retinoids in clinical use are *isotretinoin and *etretinate.

Regressions induced by retinoids have been reported recently in four cases of *skin cancer (reference in Appendix), with few side effects. *Vitamin A is the richest source of retinoids in the *diet.

To prevent changes due to ageing in the skin, retinoids have to be applied twice a day for 6 months before they have any effect, and there-after at least once a day for life. They do not reverse age-induced changes to the skin of anyone over 50 years of age. There are also temporary side-effects for most users—severe patches of redness and peeling that can last up to three months before subsiding.

Although retinoids have few serious side effects, they can cause malformations of the developing baby in the uterus and should not be used by women who may become pregnant.

riboflavin   *vitamin B2. Deficiency of this vitamin is probably not itself a factor in the development of cancer, but a *diet deficient in riboflavin is usually deficient in other vitamins, including those which may be necessary for protection against cancer. See *vitamins.

risk factors for cancer   see *causes of cancer

RNA, ribonucleic acid   is a class of compounds chemically similar to *DNA. Messenger RNA (mRNA) is a *transcript of a section of DNA, using a similar four-letter code, that contains the instructions for a cell to make a particular *protein product. mRNA acts as a template, rather like a punch card detailing instructions for a machine. The letters in the RNA code are U, C, A and G, as compared to T, C, A and G in the DNA code. Other forms of RNA take part in the joining of *amino acids to make proteins.

In some viruses, like *HIV, which is the cause of *AIDS, RNA is the hereditary informational blueprint instead of DNA. See *nature of cancer, *genetic code.

rodent ulcer   non-healing sore caused by *skin cancer of the *basal cell carcinoma type, usually in sun-exposed skin

Rous, F. Peyton   1879–1970 American scientist of the Rockefeller University of New York, who discovered that certain tumours in domestic fowls could be transmitted by invisible infectious particles, later shown to be *viruses. Unfortunately his work was not believed, and pressure from his colleagues forced him to abandon it. It is now a famous story that Rous had to wait until he was 85 years old before receiving the Nobel Prize for this work. See* viruses and cancer.

Roxby Downs   town near the *Olympic Dam mine in South Australia which produces gold, copper, silver and *uranium ores. See *atomic bombs and nuclear reactors.

Rubidomycin   trade name of daunomycin, medication used in cancer *chemotherapy

S

sarcoma   general name of a class of cancer arising in connective tissue. See *names of cancers.

Schleiden, Matthias   1804–1881 German botanist, professor in several universities in Germany and in Dorpat, Holland, whose fame rests on studies from which he concluded that all plants consist of *cells. Further, he taught that the cell was an organism in itself and that it propagated itself by means of its *nucleus. These are fundamental tenets of modern biology.

Schwann, Theodor   1810–1882, German anatomist, professor in Louvain, Belgium, who is credited with establishing by his work and publications that all plants and animals consist of *cells. He showed that cells of plants and animals were esssentially similar. In fact, others before him, including *Schleiden, had described and named cells, but history accords Schwann the honour of demonstrating by most thorough study that cells formed plants, embryos and full-grown animals.

screening for cancer   Since it has been established that the outlook in many cancers can be improved by early treatment, it is logical to attempt to diagnose all cancers early. The question is: can cancer be diagnosed before the patient is aware of symptoms? Doctors can pick up cancers earlier than patients, because they have ways of investigating and diagnosing. Should everybody avail him- or herself of these skills? Should special tests be used to screen the public *en masse*?

Everybody cannot be screened for everything. Who can be screened, and for what, depend on the frequency of the condition to be detected, the benefit of early diagnosis in the particular condition and the cost of the screening procedure.

*Malignant melanoma, cancer of the large *bowel, *breast, *skin, *head and neck are examples where early diagnosis makes an important difference in the outcome. The outlook for patients treated early for malignant melanoma is excellent. The penalty for late diagnosis is a high risk of death.

There are many unanswered questions about screening. Proof can only be obtained by properly organised prospective *clinical trials (i.e. studies that watch the differences in outcome develop between the screened and non-screened groups). Proof of this sort has not yet been obtained to show a difference in mortality between women offered teaching in *breast self-examination and comparable women who have not been taught.

A medical examination incorporates screening procedures that require no sophisticated equipment. Doctors can palpate abdomens

185

and breasts, examine skin and body orifices. Expert examination of the skin is highly effective in eliminating the dangers of *skin cancer, by dealing with precancerous changes and early cancers. A rectal examination is an excellent screening examination for cancer in the *rectum and *prostate, and will occasionally pick up other tumours in the pelvis. Rectal examination requires skill but little time and cost, and although the prospect of the examination is unpleasant, it is no more uncomfortable than passing a bowel motion.

Women should be screened regularly for cancer of the uterine *cervix. This disease is detectable by a *smear test when it is in the very earliest stage, no more than a layer of cells thick. It can then be cured without causing any lasting disturbance.

Testing bowel motions for blood has a place in the detection of *bowel cancer if done properly, but the interpretation of stool blood tests is a matter for the doctor, since even bleeding caused by harsh brushing of the teeth can be detected by tests for blood in stools, as can blood from food and from trouble anywhere in the bowel. New tests, just coming on the market and based on antibodies to human blood, offer more reliable screening for bleeding from bowel cancers.

Screening for *lung cancer is not so easy. A chest X-ray examination does not usually find lung cancers early enough. Tests for cancer cells in sputum are used to screen *uranium miners, and mass surveys are carried out in Japan on sputum—in some surveys by subjects collecting their own sputum and mailing the preparation to the laboratory.

Some types of cancer cannot be detected early by screening tests.

People who have been identified as having a particular cancer risk, for example if here is a family history of particular cancers, should be kept under the appropriate surveillance (*see heredity and cancer). Persons with bowel *polyps, *pernicious anaemia (with increased risk of stomach cancer), *bladder polyps or benign lumps in the breasts are examples of people who need surveillance.

It may be considered necessary to screen for cancers caused by carcinogens in the workplace. See *occupation and cancer.

Because of the seriousness of the problem, several governments have set up pilot programmes to assess the value of screening for *breast cancer, by breast self-examination and *mammography.

One per cent of blood donors in Japan test positive for *antibodies to the virus *HTLV-I, which is the cause of *adult T cell leukaemia. As the cancer has a 20–30 year incubation period, the disease could be spread by blood transfusion without it being detected in the recipients (for many years). HTLV-I is found sporadically outside of Japan, and some blood banks are now beginning to screen for this virus.

secondary cancer or *metastasis, tumour derived from seedlings from a *primary cancer in a different part of the body

selenium   chemical element. Deficiency of selenium may be a factor in the causation of cancer. See *mineral deficiency and cancer.

Sellafield   British nuclear power installation formerly called *Windscale. See also *atomic bombs and nuclear reactors.

seminoma   type of *testis cancer

scrotum cancer   *skin cancer occurring in chimney sweeps, caused by *tar. See also *chemicals as causes of cancer, *mineral oil.

shale oil   *see chemicals as causes of cancer

shingles   also known as herpes zoster, rash and painful eruption of the skin caused by a virus which also causes chicken pox. Shingles is a reactivation of an infection dormant since childhood chicken pox, affecting one or more nerves. The rash occurs in the area of skin served by the nerve. It can be on any part of the body, including the face. The first symptom is pain in the affected area. A rash appears up to 4 or 5 days later, which goes on to form blisters which then burst.

Herpes zoster is not uncommon in persons who are debilitated for any reason and particularly those receiving *chemotherapy. It is important to recognize the condition early, preferably before the rash is established, so the effective treatment can be given with *acyclovir. This medication, given intravenously, reduces the pain associated with the eruption and the pain which commonly persists. It also reduces the severity of the rash.

'sick office syndrome'   a set of symptoms attributed to *air pollution in poorly ventilated buildings. The symptoms are itchy eyes, irritated skin, dry throats, fatigue, running noses, headaches, nausea and coughing. These symptoms are not apparently related to cancer, but air in such buildings could contain relatively high concentrations of cancer-inducing substances.

According to a study of 10 buildings conducted by the National Aeronautics and Space Administration (NASA) and the Associated Landscape Contractors of America (ALCA), indoor air could be 100 times as polluted as outdoor air in large American industrial cities. Newer buildings are particularly prone to cause problems because they are designed to maximise energy savings. These studies suggest that current building industry standards on the amount of fresh air available per person per minute should be revised upwards from 5 to a minimum of 15 cubic feet (1.4 to 4.2 cubic metres).

The NASA/ALCA study pointed to one way of helping reduce the sick office syndrome. Plants are capable of removing low levels of pollutants such as *benzene and *formaldehyde from the air, as

Sites of cancer

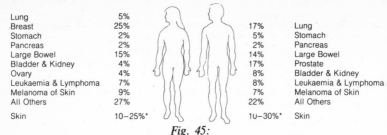

Lung	5%	17%	Lung
Breast	25%	5%	Stomach
Stomach	2%	2%	Pancreas
Pancreas	2%	14%	Large Bowel
Large Bowel	15%	17%	Prostate
Bladder & Kidney	4%	8%	Bladder & Kidney
Ovary	4%	8%	Leukaemia & Lymphoma
Leukaemia & Lymphoma	7%	7%	Melanoma of Skin
Melanoma of Skin	9%	22%	All Others
All Others	27%		
Skin	10–25%*	1∪–30%*	Skin

Fig. 45:

*Relative incidence of different types of cancer, showing the contribution each type of cancer makes to the total cancer burden, excluding non-melanoma skin cancer. For example, a relative frequency of 5% in men means that that cancer makes up 5% of all cancers in men. * = proportion having non-melanoma skin cancers. These are averages of Australian and US figures. Compare this with Fig. 22, which shows the relative mortality from the same cancers.*

shown by accumulation of these substances in the roots. The plant species they studied were *potos* (devil's ivy), *spatiphylum* (madonna lily) and philodendrons. It is hoped that the pollutants absorbed by the plants are degraded by them.

sites of cancer   Globally, cancer occurs most commonly in the *sto-mach. Cancers of the *lung, *breast, large *bowel and *cervix of the uterus follow in frequency. Cancers of the *skin, *pancreas and *ovary are also common, but worldwide estimates of their prevalence are unreliable.

In Western countries the digestive organs are the commonest sites of the internal cancers. About one quarter of all cases of cancer occur in these organs, which include the stomach, the *oesophagus (the 'gullet'), the large bowel and the pancreas. The incidence of these cancers is relatively high in both males and females. The majority of cancers of the digestive organs (amounting to 14% of cancers) occur in the large bowel, including the *rectum. Many cancers of the large bowel and rectum could be detected earlier, using available measures, and cured.

Cancer of the lung is the commonest cancer in males, causing 27% of cancer deaths. Cancers of lung account for 17% of cancers in males and 5% of cancers in females. The incidence of cancer of the lung is increasing steadily in women. As the rate of cure of cancer of the lung is low, this cancer accounts for a relatively high proportion of deaths from cancer.

The commonest cancer in females is cancer of the breast, account-ing for more than one quarter of cancers in women and about one fifth of female cancer deaths.

Other relatively common cancers are *leukaemias and *lymphomas (8% of cancers, affecting both sexes) and cancers of the *prostate (17% of cancers in men), *bladder and *uterus.

Cancers of the *skin are frequent, and curable if treated early. Other important sites of cancer are in the *head and *neck including the mouth and tongue, and the *kidneys and *brain. Tables 8 and 10, and Fig 45 show the incidence of the different cancers in people in Western societies and how frequently they cause death.

SKIN CANCER

The skin is the largest organ of the body. It is composed of two layers, an inner layer called the dermis and an outer layer called the epidermis. The hairs, sweat and oil glands, nerves and blood vessels are in the tough elastic dermis. *Stem cells of the basal layer of the epidermis multiply to produce mature cells whose function is to make the body watertight and to resist most chemical substances. As the stem cells multiply, their progeny move towards the surface, die, become compressed and eventually flake off. Pigment cells (*melano-cytes) are also located in the basal layer of the epidermis.

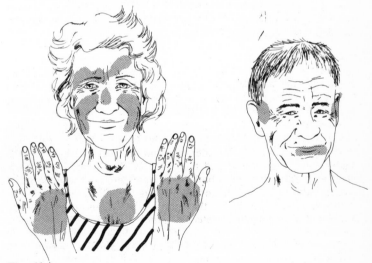

Fig. 46:

Basal cell carcinoma (left), caused by exposure to sunlight, occurs anywhere on the face and head and neck, and on the back of the hands and forearms. Squamous cell carcinoma is also related to exposure to the sun and may occur in the same places. A lump or ulcer on the lower lip is particularly likely to be a squamous cancer (right).

Skin cancer

Types of Skin Cancer

There are three main types of skin cancers. In Australia 75% are *basal cell carcinomas, 20% are *squamous cell carcinomas and most of the rest are *malignant melanomas. Malignant melanomas arise from the *melanocytes while basal and squamous cell carcinomas arise from the epidermal cells.

Australians have the highest rate of skin cancers in the world; 1 in every 60 will develop a melanoma and 2 out of 3 will develop one of the other common skin cancers. One hundred and forty thousand cases of skin cancer are treated annually, at a direct cost of $100 million. Of the 3–4000 patients with melanoma each year about 700 die, while 2000 die of other skin cancers. Melanoma and squamous cell cancers are definitely occurring more frequently.

Basal and squamous cell carcinomas occur most commonly in people over the age of 40. Malignant melanoma can occur from adolescence onward and is most common between 30 and 50 years of age. It is rare in children. The incidence of malignant melanoma is rising in Australia and other Western countries. Death rates for malignant melanoma have increased by about 150% in men and 280% in women over the last 30 years. This increase is not simply explained by the fashion for acquiring a suntan. Among men, the highest incidence in the world occurs in Queensland.

Cause of Skin Cancer

Cancer of the skin can usually be attributed to one or more factors. *Soot was the first cause of skin cancer to be recognised, causing *scrotum cancer in chimney sweeps. Today chemicals in *shale oil, including *polycyclic hydrocarbons may cause cancer in workers in some industries.

The most important factor causing skin cancer is the *ultraviolet light from the sun. Persons whose ancestors came from the British Isles, and whose skin tans poorly, are paricularly susceptible, especially if they live in very sunny climates like those of Australia and the southern US. Severe sunburn at any age, but particularly in childhood, significantly increases the risk of development of skin cancer.

Pigment in skin protects it from ultraviolet damage and subsequent cancer. In caucasians, skin cancers occur most commonly on the head, neck and arms. In negroes they occur just as frequently on unexposed areas.

Table 15: Four types of skin cancer

1	Basal cell carcinoma
2	Squamous cell carcinoma
3	Malignant melanoma
4	Kaposi's sarcoma

The body's reaction to the sun is to move pigment, called *melanin (the word is derived from the Greek word for black) to the surface of the skin to help block out ultraviolet rays. Melanin produces the bronze sun tan so desired by many, but the sun also causes skin damage and prolonged exposure results in changes to cells of the basal layer of the skin, which may lead to cancer.

Ultraviolet light damages *DNA. If this damage occurs constantly and over many years, it is only a matter of time before a faulty repair is made. Faulty repair of damaged DNA constitutes a *mutation. One of the mutations will eventually cause cancerous behaviour. People suffering from a rare disease called *xeroderma pigmentosum have a particularly high risk of developing skin cancer.

Persons whose immune defences are down, for any reason, including *chemotherapy for cancer, or similar treatments to enable them to accept kidney and other tissue grafts, have a tendency to develop skin cancers. This applies particularly to *AIDS victims. See *immunity and cancer, *medical treatment as a cause of cancer.

One of the reasons for the increase in the incidence of skin cancer is believed by some experts to be the depletion of the *ozone layer surrounding the Earth. This depletion is allowing more utlraviolet rays to reach the Earth's surface. Over the past 10 years, the incidence of skin cancers in Tasmania has doubled and the Tasmanian rates are double those of regions of similar latitude in the northern hemisphere. Tasmania is closer to the Antarctic ozone hole than any other populated place.

*Arsenic and *X-rays also cause skin cancers. Squamous cell carcinomas arise sometimes in chronic scars and ulcers. In Kashmir, cancer results on the chest, abdomen and thighs from burning by hot earthenware pots used for warming the body. Use of a loincloth in some Indian groups results in cancers in the groin, flanks and buttocks.

*Papilloma virus is usually a causative factor in *penis and *cervix cancer, which have the features of squamous cell carcinoma. Other kinds of squamous cell cancer on the skin have not been associated with papilloma virus.

South Australian figures for melanoma show an increase in beachside areas of up to 49% above the average for the State. People in upper-income suburbs have a 74% increase above the average. The inference is that those who work during the week and sunbake on the weekend, or take holidays in sunny places, are at greatest risk. Migrants to South Australia have a lower incidence of melanoma than those born in the State. The longer migrants live there, the closer their melanoma rate approaches that of the SA-born person. Since the early 1950s, the mortality rates for melanoma in that State have increased by about 140% in men and 370% in women.

*Polychlorinated biphenyls have been suspected of causing malignant melanoma.

191

Skin cancer

Skin Conditions That Precede Cancer

When *arsenic was an industrial hazard, *warts often preceded the development of a skin cancer. The skin of the hands of the first doctors to use X-rays became thin and degenerate some years before the first cancers emerged. Nowadays skin cancers, excepting perhaps melanomas, occur in skin that shows degenerative changes due to sunlight, called *solar keratoses.

A *solar keratosis is a dry, rough, firm stable spot on the skin, common in people over 40. It is not a skin cancer, but a minority may change into skin cancers, so they should be checked when they appear or when they change. Solar keratoses are an indication of sufficient exposure to the sun to develop skin cancer. Therefore, people who have developed keratoses should take particular care to protect their skins from the sun.

A thin superficial blush of dark pigment sometimes precedes development of a melanoma.

About 10% of melanomas occur in people with a condition called *dysplastic naevus syndrome. These persons have many pigmented moles (naevi) on the skin, from which melanomas may develop. They need to be watched carefully.

Basal Cell Carcinoma

Basal cell cancers usually start in the skin of the face, top of the ears, V of the neck, backs of the hands and forearms, as small round or flattened lumps. They often start in scaly patches. If untreated they frequently form ulcers (*rodent ulcers), which often appear as un-healed sores.

Basal cell carcinoma usually grows slowly, over months to years and rarely spreads to other parts of the body. It simply grows, ulcerates and destroys the surrounding tissues.

Basal cell carcinomas can be prevented by regular treatment of suspicious areas of scaly skin by freezing with liquid nitrogen, a procedure that is quick and causes little inconvenience. Treatment is by *surgery or *radiotherapy.

Squamous Cell Carcinoma

Squamous cell cancers appear on skin most often exposed to the sun, as scaling, red areas which may bleed easily and ulcerate, look-ing like an unhealing sore. They grow over weeks to months, but invade deeply and spread to other parts of the body, if neglected.

Squamous cell cancer must be diagnosed early to prevent spread to distant parts and so that the tissue, for example the lip, is not mutilated by the treatment, which may be *surgery or *radiotherapy. In the *mouth they may be very difficult to cut out when large, and the operation may require extensive plastic surgery.

*Bowen's disease is the name given to a squamous cell cancer confined to the superficial layer of the skin (the *epidermis) that

Fig. 47:

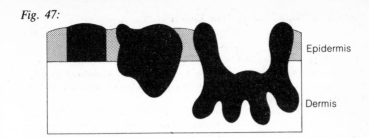

Epidermis

Dermis

Basal cell carcinoma. The first sign of basal cell carcinoma
may be a scaly patch of sun-affected skin, then a small area of skin
may become raised (left). This skin cancer commonly develops a
raised margin (centre). It often ulcerates after it has been in
existence for some time (right).

looks like a scaly patch of skin which oozes when scraped. It does not
spread until it has been present long enough to grow down into the
*dermis. Cases that arise on skin that is not exposed to the sun are
usually the result of ingestion of arsenic.

Malignant Melanoma

Malignant melanoma is relatively uncommon but dangerous. Melanomas appear as new spots, freckles or *moles which change in
colour, thickness or shape over a period of months. Often they are
dark brown to black, red or blue-black. Malignant melanoma can
appear in skin in any place in the body and occasionally in other
places than skin, wherever there is pigment. The inside of the eye is
one such place.

Early detection and treatment of malignant melanoma are essential. The possibility of cure of malignant melanoma is related directly
to the thickness of the cancer. If it has not spread down into the
underlying dermal layer, it is usually cured by *surgery. South Australian figures show survival rates of 83% for males and 91% for
females. When malignant melanoma is spread through other parts of
the body it is incurable, because it relapses after *radiotherapy or
*chemotherapy.

Everybody should know about dark skin spots. If they bleed,
become warty or change their appearance, they should be seen to
immediately.

Experts can often say from the appearance if there is cause for
concern. Often a *biopsy must be taken for microscopical examination. If a doctor is not a skin specialist or plastic surgeon, he should
not hesitate to refer the patient to an expert. Neglecting to make a
correct diagnosis may cost the patient his life.

Kaposi's Sarcoma

This skin tumour warrants mention here because it is likely to be seen with increasing frequency. Kaposi's Sarcoma occurs mostly in tropical Africa, and was otherwise seen in people of Mediterranean descent and in Ashkenazi Jews. Since about 1979, with the spread of the *AIDS epidemic, Kaposi's sarcoma has been found with increasing frequency in AIDS patients in Western populations.

It appears as painless red-purple patches on any part of the body, most noticeably on the skin. It seems that it is not the AIDS virus itself which causes Kaposi's sarcoma, but other infections which the

Table 16: Guidelines for avoiding skin cancers

---

1 Minimise sun exposure during the hours of 10 am to 2 pm (11 am to 3 pm during daylight saving time) when the sun is strongest. **The cult of sunbathing is dangerous.**

2 Keep **infants** out of the sun. Begin using *sunscreens on children at 6 months of age, then allow graduated and moderate exposure to the sun.

3 Teach children sun protection early. Sun damage occurs with each unprotected sun exposure and accumulates over the course of a lifetime.

4 Wear a **hat,** long-sleeved shirts and long pants when in the sun. Choose tightly-woven materials.

5 Apply a **sunscreen** before every exposure to the sun and reapply frequently and liberally, at least every 2 hours, while in the sun. The sunscreen should always be reapplied after swimming or perspiring heavily. Use sunscreens with an SPF (sunscreen protection factor) of 15 or more.

6 Use sunscreens even on overcast days, since the sun's rays are as damaging on cloudy, hazy days as they are on sunny days.

7 Use sunscreens at high altitudes, because there is less atmosphere to absorb the sun's rays.

8 Sand, snow, water and concrete greatly increase exposure of skin to damaging light by reflection of light.

9 Individuals whose risk of skin cancer is high (outdoor workers, fair-skinned individuals and persons who have already had skin cancer) should apply sunscreens daily.

10 Persons over 50 years, younger persons with fair, lightly pigmented skin and anybody with a suspicious spot should pay an annual visit to a dermatologist.

It is particularly important that these guidelines are accepted by families and instilled into children from an early age.

AIDS patient cannot fight. *DNA of *cytomegalovirus has been found in the tumours. Cytomegalovirus is a very common organism which only causes illness in the very young or in patients whose immune defences are weakened. See *immunity and cancer.

Kaposi's sarcoma is thought to arise in cells which line blood vessels. It usually causes multiple patches on the skin. The cancers may spread to lymph nodes, to the bowel and elsewhere.

Treatment is with *interferon, *chemotherapy and/or local *radio-therapy, but the response is not very good as a rule. The condition becomes very disfiguring and causes death by spreading to the brain, bowel and bone marrow.

Diet and Skin Cancer
There is some evidence from studies with experimental animals that *vitamins C and *E, and beta-*carotene help prevent skin cancer. An excess of *fats should be avoided. See *diet.

Warning Signs of Skin Cancer
Warning signs of cancer include changes in skin texture, particularly in moles or blemishes. Persistent small scaly patches of the sun-exposed areas must be attended to.

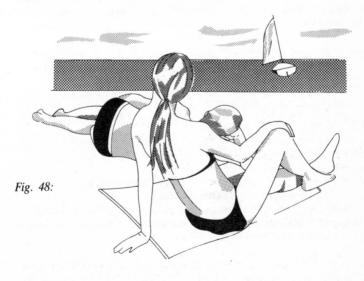

Fig. 48:

The dangerous cult of sunbathing. Enjoy it now, pay later with skin degeneration and skin cancer. Exposure to the sun's ultraviolet light in childhood is the most serious factor causing skin cancer.

Table 17: Suspicious changes in skin

1   Ulcers
2   Bleeding
3   Scaly patches
4   Changes in skin moles
Rise in height of the mole
Change in colour
A new mole
Change in size
Change in sensation
Change in shape
Change in texture

smear test   test of the *cervix of the uterus, in which cell samples are obtained by gentle wiping with a wooden spatula and a cotton bud. The process may be uncomfortable but should not be painful. The sampled cells are smeared on microscope slides for special staining ('Pap' or *Papanicolaou staining) permitting identification of abnormal cells and cancer cells. Abnormal cells may not be due to cancer; infection with various microorganisms may temporarily cause cells in the smear to appear abnormal.

smoking   *see tobacco

snuff   *see tobacco

socioeconomic class and cancer   On average, the poor have more cancer than the wealthy. This applies to many types of cancer, including cancer of the *lung and *cervix.

In general, the most financially disadvantaged people smoke more, have poorer diets and have a greater exposure to occupational carcinogens.

By contrast, the highest incidence of *bowel cancer is found in people belonging to the highest socioeconomic class. The reason is evidently a *diet rich in meats and animal *fats. The incidence of *malignant melanoma is higher in upper- and middle-socioeconomic districts. See *causes of cancer.

solar keratosis   scaly, firm skin spot arising in persons who have had long exposure to sunlight. A proportion, probably small, of these spots, develops into *skin cancer.

soot   see *polycyclic hydrocarbons

Spiess, Heinz b 1920, German paediatrician, professor in Munich, who showed that radium-224 caused bone cancers. See *radiation.

sperm banking preservation of spermatozoa by storage at very low temperatures. Potentially valuable in *testis cancer.

squamous cell carcinoma see *skin cancer

stem cell population of cells within those tissues which can regrow, such as skin, blood and bowel, that gives rise to new cells. Stem cells have the remarkable property of producing unlike progeny. Every time a stem cell divides one daughter cell goes on to mature and carry out the work of the tissue; the other remains behind as a stem cell.

Cancers arise in stem cells. See *nature of cancer.

stoma an opening, name given to the opening of the bowel on the abdominal wall when a *colostomy has been created. See also *bowel cancer.

STOMACH CANCER

The stomach is a reservoir holding food immediately after it has been swallowed.

Cause of Cancer of the Stomach

The mortality from stomach cancer has been declining in many countries in the past 30 years, although the reasons for this decrease have not been identified. Japan has about 25 times more stomach cancer than those Western countries with the lowest incidence. Better preservation of food, using refrigeration and other non-chemical means, has possibly played a part, as has reduced consumption of salt-cured food. Refrigeration also reduces contamination by bacteria and fungi, and makes it possible to eat more fruit.

Certainly, stomach cancer accompanies a low standard of living. In the United States, Great Britain and Australia, where the incidence is already low, the fall in stomach cancer is greater in younger people. This is thought to show that changes of recent years, whatever they may be, are reducing the risk still further. A study of Greek migrants to Australia has shown that they have less stomach cancer than they would have had in Greece.

Apart from the presumed contamination of food, *pernicious anaemia, which is treated with vitamin B_{12} injections, is a risk factor for cancer of the stomach. More than 10 years ago, before good medications were available to treat ulcers of the stomach and duodenum, many ulcer patients were treated by partial removal of their stomachs. These patients have an increased risk of developing stomach cancer and they should undergop regular *endoscopy. One

Stomach cancer

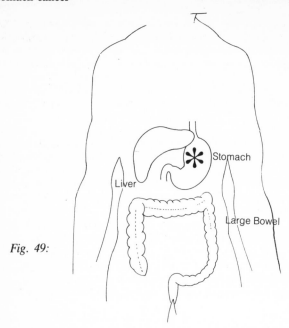

Fig. 49:

Cancer of the stomach. Food passes from the mouth through the oesophagus or gullet to the stomach. Cancer of the stomach (*) is now a relatively infrequent cancer in Western countries and its incidence appears to be declining.

study suggests that adequate *vitamin A in the diet halves the risk of stomach cancer.

Ulcers are relatively common in the stomach, but cancer rarely develops in the common type of ulcer. Sometimes an ulcer that was thought to be *benign proves to be a cancer. For this reason, it is good practice when an ulcer is first diagnosed to make sure that it heals with treatment. If it does not, a *biopsy should be taken.

Symptoms of Stomach Cancer

Cancer of the stomach may present itself to the patient as abdominal pain, loss of appetite, 'indigestion'—discomfort after meals—or loss of blood from the stomach. Sudden bleeding from a cancer usually causes the patient to vomit blood. The patient who vomits blood will almost always think of cancer, and it is always a sign of a serious condition, although the cause is much more commonly a benign ulcer than a cancer.

Slower bleeding results in loss in the bowel motions and the patient develops *anaemia, which causes tiredness and shortness of breath.

The blood undergoes partial digestion, causing the bowel motions to become dark, usually black. The chance finding of anaemia or of blood in the motions is sometimes the first indication of stomach cancer.

Indigestion or other symptoms in patients who have pernicious anaemia are an indication for examination of the stomach through a flexible *gastroscope.

Treatment of Cancer of the Stomach

Cancer of the stomach is only curable if it is diagnosed early. It soon spreads locally, becoming inoperable, and to other organs, particularly the liver. *Chemotherapy and *radiotherapy are disappointing in the treatment of incurable stomach cancer. An operation may be carried out in incurable cases as a symptomatic measure, to provide a passage for food.

Prevention of Cancer of the Stomach

A good diet with fresh food and plenty of fruit is an obvious measure for the prevention of stomach cancer.

In Japan, where cancer of the stomach is relatively common, screening campaigns are carried out by introducing cameras into the stomach. Screening is not feasible in most Western countries. Patients who have abdominal complaints should seek medical advice.

stress, psychological factors and mental illness From antiquity, mental shocks, melancholia or depression and *bereavement have been thought to bring on cancer. The evidence for these beliefs is very slender, but perhaps they should not be discarded until more work is done.

The major problem in showing a connection between the state of mind and the induction of cancer is the difficulty in providing valid evidence. Studies have been published purporting to show a connection between the type of personality that is involved both in smoking and the development of cancer.

It has been proposed that married, single and divorced men have differing risks of dying from cancer. Married men have the best risk, divorced men the worst, and risk for single men is intermediate. Divorced men tend also to have a poorer *diet, to drink more *alcohol and to smoke more *tobacco.

Can the state of mind influence the course of cancer? Many believe it can. Many patients declare that they are going to beat cancer by adopting a positive attitude. A recent study, carried out with great care to avoid bias and errors, concluded that psychosocial intervention enhanced the survival of a group of patients with advanced *breast cancer. The psychological treatment consisted of group therapy led by a psychiatrist or social worker, with a therapist who had had breast cancer, meeting weekly for 90 minutes.

strontium-90   radioactive element, having a *half-life of 29.1 years, released in nuclear accidents. Strontium-90 is incorporated into bones in place of calcium and remains in them for many years. See *atomic bombs and nuclear accidents.

Sun Protection Factor (SPF) number   see *sunscreens

sunscreens   lotions, gels, sprays and lipsticks which protect the skin against damaging effects of the sun's rays. They contain chemicals which absorb, reflect or scatter *ultraviolet light.

Sunscreens can greatly reduce, but not totally prevent, skin damage. Sun protection factor (SPF) is a measure of the protective capacity of sun-screens, determined by the Australian Standards Association and indicated on the product label.

The SPF numbers range from 2 to 15. SPF 15 or 15+ gives maximum protection. The protection also depends on the skin type; people with reddish or fair hair are still most susceptible even with sunscreen, people with dark hair and skin burn least, and those with light brown hair have intermediate susceptibility to sun damage.

It is important that the sunscreen should also be labelled 'BROAD SPECTRUM', to be sure of protection from all *ultraviolet light (UVA and UVB). See *skin cancer.

surgery   Surgery is the correction of bodily disorders by cutting, joining and removal of tissues. Every surgical operation therefore involves damage to tissues, which calls forth a reaction by the body and requires bodily repair processes. There is usually some pain postoperatively, which should be well controlled by proper management.

Most operations require anaesthesia, which may be local or general. To achieve local anaesthesia, sensation can be cut off from parts of the body by temporarily blocking pain messages to the brain. Local anaesthesia involves application of anaesthetising medication, usually by injection, but also by spray to mucous membranes or by ointment.

General anaesthesia stops the appreciation of pain by temporarily interrupting brain activity. General anaesthesia is commenced by giving an injection, after which the patient has no consciousness of events until after the operation. Modern anaesthetics have overcome the problem of *nausea and the patient usually experiences few ill effects.

Surgery today is enormously safter than it was even a few decades ago, but every surgical operation involves some risk. There are side effects of anaesthesia and surgery and each patient must be assessed for fitness to undergo the proposed procedure. Account must be taken of the general fitness, the other illnesses which they may have and whatever medications they are taking.

The reactions of the body to surgery may cause fever and *pain postoperatively. These risks include postoperative infections, heart troubles, respiratory difficulties, bleeding, clot formation and disturbances of body chemistry and fluid balance.

The risks of surgery are obviously greater if the patient has important pre-existing medical problems like high blood pressure, heart disease, diabetes and lung problems. The risks also depend on who does the operation and where it is done. Everybody has the right to choose a surgeon he or she believes to be highly skilled in the particular operation and to undergo the operation in a good centre. The more serious the operations, the more important it is for the surgery to be carried out in a centre specialising in the particular operation. One criterion of excellence is whether the surgeon is engaged in or associated with a centre that is engaged in research and teaching, for example, a university teaching hospital. Another essential is the availability of doctors and equipment for the management of complications that may arise during or after the operation.

In deciding whether or not to recommend a particular operation for a cancer patient, the advantages and disadvantages will be weighed carefully. If the operation offers a chance of cure, or if operation offers a better chance of cure than other treatments, the risks that are taken may have to be bigger than would be acceptable for an operation to palliate. All these things must be discussed with the surgeon and the cancer team. Every patient has the right to full and informed explanations and the doctors have the responsibility to provide these.

All patients also have the right to seek another opinion before committing themselves to an operation.

Early surgery cures a high proportion of all cancers of the *skin and *bowel. Surgery offers a chance of cure of tumours of *lung, *stomach, *breast, *uterus, *ovary, *testis and many other less common tumours. Surgical removal of a tumour fails to cure the cancer if cells from the tumour have already spread to other parts of the body.

Surgery may be needed to treat the complications of cancer. Sometimes the bowel is obstructed, or the spinal cord is compressed. Surgery is often part of the plan of treatment even when the cancer cannot be cured, because it controls unpleasant or painful symptoms. See *treatment.

Sydenham, Thomas 1624–1689, celebrated English physician, sometimes called 'the English Hippocrates'. Hippocrates of Cos, 470–375 BC, has been called the 'father of medicine'. Sydenham wrote on the use of morphine to control *pain.

symptom any noticeable discomfort or disturbance of health or wellbeing. Symptoms are the complaints the patient describes to the doctor, as contrasted to signs a doctor may find on examination of the patient.

T

2,4,5-T *organochlorine herbicide, component of *Agent Orange, widely used throughout the world, but no longer manufactured, at least in the USA. 2,4,5-T is not known to cause cancer in humans. 2,4,5-T is always contaminated by *dioxins.

tamoxifen medication used to treat *breast cancer. Tamoxifen is an inhibitor of *oestrogen. It is a very safe drug, with few side effects. As it inhibits oestrogen it may cause hot flushes, and mild uterine bleeding. It may cause nausea during the first few days of treatment, for which reason it is usual to start with half the treatment dose. By cutting off the body's supply of oestrogen tamoxifen may worsen the thinning of bones that occurs in women after the menopause. See *chemotherapy.

tannin, tannic acid terms for a class of astringent substances in a variety of plant preparations, including *tea and wine. *Tannins in adequate concentration precipitate *proteins, damage membranes of the stomach and bowel and the liver. There seems, however, to be no cause for concern about the ordinary consumption of tannins in tea and wine.

tar dark brown or viscous material obtained from coal or wood. Similar materials arise when other substances are burnt. Tar contains many *carcinogens. *Creosote is a carcinogenic product of tar. See *chemicals as causes of cancer, *occupation and cancer.

tea universal beverage. There is no good evidence that tea causes cancer. *Tannin in the tea has been implicated, but the evidence is not strong. There is far more danger to tea drinkers from *tobacco smoke and studies have not been able to disprove that cancers occurring in tea drinkers are due to smoking.
Herbal teas are another matter and are best avoided. They are not standard preparations and some are undoubtedly toxic. Herbal teas also contain tannins in relatively high concentration.

television screens and video display units Concern has been expressed from time to time about television screens and video display terminals of computers (VDUs). Rays from television screens have a very short penetration in air. Pregnancies in mice exposed to the same radiation were not affected by it. Studies have suggested that women using video display terminals may suffer more anxiety, depression and menstrual problems than co-workers not using terminals, but no good evidence has been gathered to suggest that the risk of cancer is significant.

TESTIS CANCER

One per cent of tumours of men occur in the testes and figures from Britain show a doubling of the incidence of testicular cancers in the 15–44 year age group during the past twenty years. They are the most frequent cancers in males between the ages of 20–35 years.

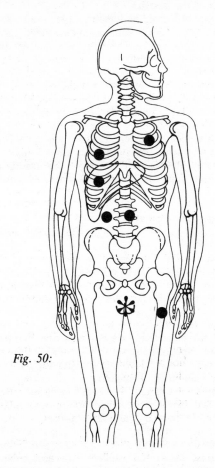

Fig. 50:

Cancer of the testis. This cancer is the most frequent in males between the ages of 20–35 years. Early diagnosis leads to a high chance of cure. In recent years, more advanced testis cancers have been cured by chemotherapy. *Testicular cancer (*) spreads to lymph nodes in the abdomen, to the lungs, to the liver and to other sites such as the bones.*

Testis cancer

There are two main types of cancer of the testis, **seminoma** and **non-seminoma (teratocarcinoma).**Both occur most frequently in young men and start as a painless lump. Both types spread to lymph glands in the abdomen and to other organs.

Cause of Cancer of the Testis

The testes are formed in the abdomen and descend during foetal life into the scrotum. A person with an undescended testis has an increased risk of testicular cancer. This risk is not completely reversed by surgical correction of the condition. In persons who had an undescended testis, as many as one fifth of the cancers occur in the normal, descended testis. This suggests that the cancer is not caused by the failure of the testis to descend, but rather that whatever causes failure of the testis to descend also influences the development of the cancer.

The incidence of testicular cancer in black men is low, suggesting that genetic factors play some part in the causation of this cancer. The environment probably plays a part too, since the incidence rises in Chinese and Japanese living in Western countries, where the risk is high.

Symptoms of Testicular Cancer

Patients notice either pain or swelling. Often the tumour is quite big before it is noticed.

Some authorities strongly recommend self-examination of the testes, particularly by men of an age in which most cancers of the testis occur, because removal of an early cancer usually cures the patient, without the need for chemotherapy or radiotherapy.

Treatment of Testicular Cancer

The first step is to remove the affected testis by *surgery. Seminoma is one of the cancers most sensitive to *radiotherapy. Seminoma patients usually receive low-dose radiotherapy to the lymph nodes of the lower abdomen. Depending on the extent of spread, non-seminoma patients are treated by surgery with or without *chemotherapy. There is debate about the need to remove lymph nodes in the lower abdomen. During such a surgical procedure, nerve branches are cut, with the result that sexual function may be impaired. The capacity for normal ejaculation may be lost. See *impotence.

Testicular tumours, like other cancers, are best treated early. However, great advances in *chemotherapy of testicular tumours have resulted in high cure rates even in advanced cases. To obtain the benefit of these advances, the treatment should be carried out by specialists working in centres for the treatment of this kind of cancer, where the best results are obtained.

Testicular cancers often produce substances which can be detected in the bloodstream. Measurement of these is valuable in showing a response to treatment and a rise in the blood level may herald a recurrence.

Sexual Function in Patients with Cancer of the Testis
Loss of fertility is a concern for patients with testicular cancer. Modern chemotherapy does not permanently disturb production of sperms. The sperm cell count decreases during the first year and normal production resumes in the second year. The healthy testis is also affected by scattered radiotherapy beams during treatment to the abdomen. Low sperm counts can be reversed by modern medications enabling most patients to father children. Sometimes the techniques of in vitro fertilization need to be used. See *infertility.

*Sperm banking should be considered before beginning treatment. However, decreased sperm cell counts, which are common before treatment, make sperm banking possible for only a minority of patients who have cancer of the testis. For most patients the best chance is proper management after the cancer is treated. At least 60% of testicular cancer patients who want to father a child are able to do so after their treatment.

For most patients, removal of one testicle does not lead to major disturbance of their sex lives by reducing sexual interest, libido or erectile potency. Some patients do develop psychological distress, coupled with impairment of sexual activity.

thorium-232 radioactive element formerly used in the X-ray contrast medium *Thorotrast for obtaining X-ray pictures of blood vessels. The half-life of thorium 228 is more than ten thousand million years. Thorotrast caused cancers of the *liver and other tissues. The liver tumours appeared an on average 19 years after administration of the Thorotrast.

Thorotrast material used before 1950 for X-ray studies of blood vessels. See *thorium-232.

Three Mile Island site of a nuclear reactor accident in USA. See *atomic bombs and nuclear reactors

thrush white spots usually at the back of the mouth or in the vagina, caused by the fungus *Candida albicans*, commonly in persons whose immunity is suppressed by *chemotherapy or *cortisone.

thyroid cancer This uncommon cancer presents as a lump or soreness in the thyroid gland, which is in the front of the neck, surrounding the front of the windpipe.

Thyroid cancer is often cured by *surgery. Some of these cancers retain the thyroid gland's capacity to take up iodine for the production of thyroid hormone. When tumours of this type have spread to other organs, the *metastases can be treated with *radio-iodine.

tissue an organised group of *cells, forming an organ or functional part of the body

tongue cancer see *head and neck cancer

TOBACCO

A surgeon, Alton *Ochsner, noticed the association between smoking and lung cancer in men who had served in World War I. Several reports came out in the 1930s and 1940s linking smoking with lung cancer, but it was not until 1950 that the irrefutable epidemiolgoical proof was obtained showing that smoking causes cancer. See *epidemiolgoical studies.

Tobacco is, in fact, the most important single *carcinogen. The world annual production of tobacco exceeds 5 million tonnes. Experts attribute 30% of cancer deaths to tobacco, which is therefore the major avoidable cause of cancer. Not only does it cause cancer of the lung, but it contributes to causation of *larynx, mouth, oesophagus, bladder, cervix, kidney and pancreas cancers.

A man who smokes heavily has roughly a 10% chance of dying of lung cancer. Heavy smokers have a greater than 20-fold risk of dying from lung cancer than non-smokers. *Air pollution increases the risk for smokers living in big cities. Smoking is extraordinarily dangerous for *uranium or *asbestos miners: the risks due to uranium and asbestos in association with smoking are not simply added, but multiplied. The same is thought to apply to other occupational carcinogens, and this is particularly serious because the populations at greatest risk from occupational exposure to carcinogens tend to have the highest smoking rates. See *occupation and cancer.

Awareness of the hazards of inhalation of other people's tobacco smoke has increased greatly of late. *Passive smoking increases the risks of lung cancer and cancer of the cervix.

So-called **smokeless tobacco** chewed or used as snuff, is just as dangerous as smoking, causing cancer where it comes into contact with gums or nasal passages. This is seen in India, where cancer of the *mouth is frequent. There, young people chew tobacco and powdered tobacco is rubbed on teeth.

The Carcinogens in Tobacco Smoke

Tobacco smoke contains literally dozens of compounds that can cause cancer. These include *polycyclic hydrocarbons, *nitrosamines, *benzene, *formaldehyde, *vinyl chloride, *arsenic, *nickel, *cadmium and the radioactive heavy metal *polonium-210.

During the past 20 years the amount of both *nicotine and *tar delivered in cigarettes has decreased by more than 50 per cent. Statistically, the use of low tar cigarettes reduces the cancer risk of smoking, but compared with not smoking or giving up, the benefits are minimal.

Cigar and pipe smokers usually inhale less smoke than cigarette smokers, and have less risk of lung cancer, although it is now clear that the risk can be just as great if the smoker inhales strongly. Cigarette, cigar and pipe smokers have about the same death rates from carcinoma of the *mouth, *larynx and *oesophagus.

The Fight against Smoking

Control of this carcinogen would be the single biggest blow in the fight against cancer.

There are two parts to the fight; preventing young people from taking up the habit and helping those who want to give it up. For both, effective action has to be based on sound principles. Public opinion and political action will decide the issue of prevention, and public education is the main strategy. At this stage, influencing public opinion is at best an art. To make education strategies more efficient, knowledge must be obtained by rigorous scientific enquiries into educational processes, political science and addiction.

*Addiction to nicotine has physical and psychological components, similar to the effects of and behavioural responses to *heroin, *morphine and *alcohol. These drugs have a similar effect on the brain. They all induce dependence and tolerance, as well as producing pleasant effects, changes of mood and cravings.

Giving up Smoking

Many experts believe that the best chance of stopping is to cease abruptly. Cutting down gradually is much less likely to work. During the weeks following cessation, abstainers need emotional support and tobacco substitutes. Various stratagems are recommended: telling all your friends, taking bets, granting personal rewards such as a year's cash value of the foregone cigarettes. Without real determination, there is little chance of success.

A person who has given up smoking will crave cigarettes for weeks and months afterwards.

Many people worry about gaining weight when they stop smoking. This is likely because tobacco suppresses appetite and reduces the efficiency of the bowel to absorb food. Food will taste better and eating can be substituted for tobacco as a reward. The solution is to avoid junk foods, to limit meals to three a day and to alter the diet if the weight starts to climb.

Many *Anti-cancer Foundations offer help and support to persons giving up smoking.

Governmental, Community and Public Health Measures

Governments cannot evade their responsibilities indefinitely. When it comes to decisions about the use of resources to defeat cancer, the best value for money would be obtained by fighting smoking. Governmental actions against tobacco require political courage, because of the effects on vested interests, revenue and employment. Many governments have acted against smoking by regulating advertising. At least one government has replaced tobacco industry financing of sporting bodies by funding from a tobacco levy. The Australian Government has banned the importation and sale of so-called smoke-less tobacco, a timely move before a dependent public has arisen.

Inevitably the tobacco industry replies to proposed legislation with advertisements, denying the health hazards associated with the use of tobacco and inciting fear of government action, particularly the restriction of the rights and freedoms of the individual.

Strategies for reducing the use of tobacco use have to focus on introduction of smoking to young people, especially girls. The fight against smoking must commit the public to deeply felt attitudes against the habit. Views are formed by using memorable ways of expression, for example 'Smoking is a slow form of suicide'. The difficulty is that the effects of smoking are delayed. People who began smoking in the 1950s are now entering the age at which lung cancer develops.

toluidine (ortho-toluidine)   chemical used in the dye industry, causing tumours of the bladder in rats and suspected of being a carcinogen. See *occupation and cancer.

translocation   abnormal rearrangement of chromosomes occurring during cell division, caused by faulty rejoining after tangling and breaking of two chromosomes. Translocation is one form of *mutation. See *nature of cancer.

transcript   An RNA transcript is a copy of a gene in *RNA code, used as a template by cells to specify the order of coupling of particular *amino acids into a *protein. See *nature of caner.

transcription   a term used to signify the copying of a gene into *RNA.

translation   the process of coupling *amino acids in the order specified by an *RNA transcript to make a *protein

trihalomethanes   *organochlorine chemicals, for example *chloroform, formed on chlorination of *water. Trihalomethanes cause liver tumours in mice.

treatment of cancer   The aim of cancer treatment is to *cure if at all possible. If cancer cannot be cured, the aim is to control the disease and palliate the *symptoms.

Cure usually requires *surgery to remove the cancer completely. Attempts at cure fail if its is not possible to remove the cancer.

Removal is not possible if the tumour has spread widely, particularly if the cancer has spread to a vital organ, such as the liver, lungs or brain. *Lasers are new tools in surgery.

*Radiotherapy (the use of X-rays in treatment), may be curative in certain situations, for example in cancer of the *skin and in early cancer of the *lung. Some cancers are cured by *chemotherapy with anticancer medications.

Virtually every kind of cancer should be treated by one or more specialists. Cancer physicians specialize in diagnosis and chemotherapy and coordinate special treatments. Cancer surgeons specialize in cancer of particular parts of the body. Radiotherapists direct X-ray treatment.

Cancer is often best treated by teams of doctors and health professionals. In major medical centres, particularly those which are associated with medical schools, specialists collaborate in cancer centres.

Cancer centres offer patients contact with specialists who are in touch with the latest trends, usually through their own participation in research.

Often the first decisions are crucial to the patient's chances of cure, or long survival. In a good team, the initial treatment is planned by the specialists who deal with particular groups of cancers. From the beginning, surgeons may need to work with radiotherapists and physicians specializing the the treatment of cancer.

tumour a general term for a swelling. Tumours may be caused by inflammations, *benign new growths such as *warts, or cancers.

U

ulcerative colitis chronic inflammatory disease of the large bowel. See *bowel cancer.

ultrasound imaging technique of mapping reflected sound waves to obtain a picture of internal organs

ultraviolet light The sun emits *electromagnetic radiation over a wide range of wavelengths. Ultraviolet (UV) light rays from the sun are invisible, of wavelength 4–400 nm. The shortest wavelengths that reach the surface of the earth through the atmosphere are about 286–290 nm. Wavelengths shorter than 286 nm are principally absorbed by *ozone in the stratosphere. In our sunlight the UV region extends from 290 to 400 nm. Rays from 400 to 760 nm are visible and perceived as colours of the rainbow from violet to red.

For practical purposes, UV rays are divided into UVA (320–400nm), UVB (290–320 nm) and UVC (shorter than 290 nm). The body needs enough exposure to UVB to make *vitamin D, which is formed when ultraviolet light in this waveband changes substances in the skin so that they can be used to make the vitamin.

UVB rays cause sunburn and subsequent skin damage, and are possibly the more dangerous in inducing skin cancers. UVA rays also damage skin tissues and can cause reactions to certain medications. *Sunscreens should be labelled 'BROAD SPECTRUM' to indicate that they block out both.

UVC is germicidal and used for sterilization.

The amount and type of solar radiation on any day depends on the latitude, time of day, the altitude and the local atmospheric conditions. Smog, smoke, dust, fog, humidity, and aerosol particles and, most importantly, the state of the ozone layer determine the amount of UV rays reaching the ground.

Since UV light does not penetrate tissue more than a few millimetres, the damage it causes is confined to the skin. UV light damages the genetic material *DNA.

*Melanin, the brown pigment of the skin, protects against the damage caused by UV light. Fair-skinned people, particularly redheads, are more susceptible than dark-skinned people to the damaging effects of UV light. These damaging effects result in both rapid ageing of the skin and in increased incidence of skin cancers.

People who work indoors and are exposed to sunlight during weekend recreation are at greater risk than outdoor workers. Exposure during childhood is thought to be extremely important in the later development of skin cancer. Migrants from England who arrived in Australia in adolescence have a lower incidence of skin cancer in adulthood than native-born Australians.

Although the precise reasons for this sensitivity to sunlight in childhood are unknown, protection from Australian sunlight during childhood reduces the rates of skin cancer of all types during the rest of life.

uranium radioactive element, breaking down to *radium. Uranium miners are at risk of developing *lung cancer, particularly if they smoke *tobacco. See *occupation and cancer, *radiation.

urethra tube-like organ draining the bladder

UTERUS (ENDOMETRIUM) CANCER
The lining of the uterus is called the *endometrium. Cancer of the endometrium is usually a disease of women after the menopause. Only 5% of cases of endometrial cancer occur before the age of 40 and 75% occur after menopause.

Cause of Cancer of the Endometrium
The risk of developing cancer of the endometrium is greater in obese women, women with high blood pressure or those who have had various menstrual irregularities.

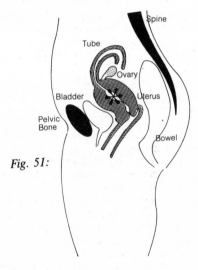

Fig. 51:

Cancer of the uterus (endometrium). Cancer of the body of the uterus arises in the layer of cells lining the cavity of the uterus, the endometrium. This cancer occurs most commonly after the menopause and usually comes to notice by uterine blood loss.

Uterus (endometrium) cancer

Symptoms of Cancer of the Endometrium
This cancer usually shows its presence by causing blood loss from the uterus. In women who are still menstruating, the warning signs may be irregular or heavy menstruation, or a watery vaginal discharge. It is essential that any postmenopausal bleeding is investigated by examination of endometrial tissue obtained by curettage.

Diagnosis of Cancer of the Endometrium
The diagnosis is made by microscopic examination of material curetted from the cavity of the uterus.

Treatment of Cancer of the Endometrium
The treatment of cancer of the uterus is *hysterectomy in early cases and surgery combined with *radiotherapy if the cancer has spread to the cervix. If carried out early, the patient has a good chance of cure. If the disease is not treated early, it spreads beyond the uterus to involve the ureters (the tubes bringing urine from the kidneys to the bladder) and other organs in the pelvis. *Radiotherapy is needed for such patients.

Some advanced cases respond to treatment with *oestrogens and *progestins, but *chemotherapy is usually disappointing.

Oral Contraceptives, Hormone Replacement and Cancer of the Uterus
Combined oral contraceptives, containing both *oestrogen and *progestin give protection against the development of endometrial carcinoma, This protection persists for some years after they have been discontinued. On the other hand, it appears that women who take unopposed oestrogens after the menopause are more likely to develop this cancer and the risk depends on how long the oestrogen is taken. The risk is probably decreased if hormones are taken in cycles.

Some authorities advise endometrial sampling before any sex hormone replacement and at intervals thereafter. Samples of endometrium may be obtained in the clinic, without anaesthesia, using special equipment.

V

vaccine   from Latin *vacca* = cow, term which stems from the use of cowpox to protect aganst the deadly smallpox virus (vaccinia virus), by Edward *Jenner in 1796. The World Health Organisation's campaign with smallpox vaccine has apparently eradicated the disease from the globe. The last recorded case of smallpox occurred in Somalia in 1977. The term vaccine today designates a preparation used for immunising against an infectious disease.

Recombinant *hepatitis B vaccine, a product of *genetic engineering, is in widespread use. This is expected to prevent *liver cancer in countries where this disease occurs frequently.

By means of genetic engineering, it is theoretically possible to make compound vaccines,. For example, *genes from a deadly virus, say poliomyelitis, could be put into the vaccinia virus, to make a compound vaccine which will safely immunise against two diseases. The use of selected genes allows the vaccinated person to build up an immunity without having to experience the toxic products of the microorganism, for example the poisons of poliomyelitis that cause paralysis.

It would be possible, for instance, to make a vaccine that contains *hepatitis B, human *papilloma virus and *Epstein-Barr virus. One vaccine would then protect against three kinds of cancer—cancer of the *liver, *Burkitt's lymphoma and cancer of the *cervix.

Vaccination will not work if the *immune system is incapable of responding. This is what happens in *AIDS, because the AIDS virus (HIV) enters key cells of that system and paralyses them. A new approach to this is to include the gene for the growth factor *interleukin-2 in the vaccine. When the weakened cells of the immune system encounter the foreign substance they are also supplied with the growth factor they need to make a response.

vagina cancer   rare cancer that occurred in women whose mothers were treated for impending miscarriage with the *oestrogen *diethrylstilboestrol, while they were in the womb.

Velban   trade name of vincristine, medication used in cancer *chemotherapy

video display units   see *television screens

vinblastine   medication used in cancer *chemotherapy

vincristine   medication used in cancer *chemotherapy

vinyl chloride   chemical used in the manufacture of plastics. Exposure to vinyl chloride monomer, the unprocessed material, caused an unusual type of *liver cancer in workers who were highly exposed to it. There is no risk from the finished product. See *chemicals as causes of cancer.

Virchow, Rudolf   1821–1902, with justification called the 'father of pathology'. Virchow brought together knowledge of abnormalities of the tissues in disease states, as studied in the mortuary and under the microscope, and the symptoms and signs of illness studied in the clinic. Among his many discoveries was the recognition of *leukaemia. He recognized the cell as the unit of all tissues and contributed to the modern understanding of cancer as an abnormality of cellular proliferation.

VIRUSES AND CANCER
It was many years before new techniques and the lessons learnt from animal studies could be used to prove that viruses cause some human cancers. Viruses are the smallest microorganisms, largely composed of genetic material *DNA or *RNA. As they do not have the complete equipment for fully independent life, viruses have to live and multiply in other *cells.

Animal Viruses and Cancer
In 1910, Peyton *Rous showed an infectious agent in extracts of tumours from **domestic fowls.** Injection of the extract caused a tumour to develop in another fowl. We now know the extract contained a tumour-causing virus.

*Warts are caused by *papilloma viruses. Warts are *benign tumours, which do not cause destruction of surrounding tissues or the death of the host. Common warts rarely become *malignant in humans.

Warts in rabbits can be transmitted by injecting an extract of warts from American cottontail rabbits. Treatment of the skin of infected rabbits with a number of *chemical carcinogens can cause some of the warts to become cancers. Studies have shown why it can be difficult to find a virus in cancers. When cancers develop, the wart virus becomes locked inside the tumour cells, and can no longer be transmitted to other rabbits or obtained in the free state. Similarly, the human *papilloma virus is locked into cancers of the *cervix. Viruses in these cancers can still be detected by *gene probing.

In 1936 *Bittner found that breast cancer was spread in some strains of mice by a virus in mothers' milk. Study of this animal cancer showed that there could be a hereditary factor in the susceptibility to cancer, because the virus did not cause cancer in some strains. Secondly, a virus can be transmitted to a young animal, but the cancer will only develop when the animal matures, because the development of this type of cancer requires the action of *oestrogen. Removal of the ovaries prevents tumours from developing, proving the requirement for female hormones in the development of these tumours. Oestrogen is also essential for the development of human breast cancers.

Studies of other animal viruses have shown that in some cases infection will only lead to cancer if it is acquired in early life, before the body's defence mechanisms are mature. *Leukaemia of cats can occur when feline leukaemia virus is introduced into households with a large number of cats. Kittens are susceptible, because they are too immature to make antibodies against the virus. Older cats protect themselves against the development of these cancers by making *antibodies that neutralize the virus.

In some cases virally-induced tumours can be prevented by making a specific *vaccine. A virus causing *lymphoma in domestic fowls, a disease that has caused disastrous losses in the chicken industry, was discovered in the 1940s. The *avian lymphoma virus is transmitted either from generation to generation through eggs, or by sick young chickens to healthy young chickens. A vaccine developed in the 1950s successfully protects against this cancer, with enormous economic benefits.

Viruses in Human Cancer

Proof of an association between a particular virus and a specific cancer had to wait until tests were developed that would identify the virus. A person's encounters with a range of viruses can be detected by measuring *antibodies in the blood, but antibodies alone are not proof that the virus had anything to with the cancer. In the last decade, teams working with Robert *Gallo in America and Luc *Montagnier in France developed ways of detecting the *human immunodeficiency virus (HIV) which causes *AIDS, while *Gissmann of Heidelberg developed *gene probing techniques for detecting human *papilloma viruses in cells of the uterine cervix. Subsequent discoveries allow the most minute quantities of virus material to be detected.

Cancers believed to be caused by viruses are listed in Table 18. Cancer viruses appear not to cause human cancers by themselves. Other co-factors are almost certainly involved, including *diet, *heredity, additional infections and various *carcinogens such as *tobacco smoke. Inability to make protective antibodies against viruses also leads to human cancers. Immune deficiency allows cancers to develop in victims of AIDS and in people whose immune system is weakened by disease or by medical treatment. See *immunity and cancer.

Vitamins

Table 18: Viruses involved in causing human cancers

Virus	Type of Cancer
Epstein-Barr virus	*Burkitt's lymphoma *nasopharyngeal carcinoma
hepatitis B virus	primary *liver cancer
papilloma virus	cancer of *cervix cancer of *penis
HTLV-I	*adult T cell leukaemia
HTLV-II	*hairy cell leukaemia
HIV (plus other agent)	*Kaposi's sarcoma *lymphoma *chronic myeloid leukaemia sundry cancers

VITAMINS

Vitamins, necessary for a number of vital chemical processes, must be included in the diet, because the body does not make them. Vitamins are divided into two broad groups: those that will dissolve in water and those that will dissolve in fat. Vitamin C and the B group vitamins are water-soluble. Vitamins A, D, E and K are fat-soluble.

Deficiencies of fat-soluble vitamins A and E have been implicated in the development of cancer. **Vitamin A**, also known as retinol, is essential for normal growth of epithelial cells, that is, cells lining body surfaces. Deficiency of this vitamin causes dry scaly skin. Vitamin A is thought to stop development of cancer and it may stop cancers progressing. The deficiency must be severe and prolonged before cancer occurs. Cancer can be induced more readily by *chemicals, viruses and *radiation in experimental animals deprived of vitamin A. *Oesophagus, *lung, *bladder and *larynx cancers have been attributed to a deficiency of vitamin A. See *retinoids.

The body obtains vitamin A in food as the fully formed vitamin and also makes the vitamin from *carotenes. The best source of these is liver, but eggs, milk products, dark green vegetables, yellow-orange vegetables and fruits are good sources. Vitamin A, like all vitamins, is best absorbed from natural sources. High doses of vitamin A capsules can be very toxic.

Vitamin B: This is a group of water-soluble substances essential for health. Deficiency of **vitamin B2** or riboflavin is not directly implicated in the causation of cancer, but a diet low in riboflavin is likely to be low in other vitamins.

Vitamin B12 is necessary for production of blood cells and is not deficient in most diets. In *pernicious anaemia, which is associated

216

Table 19: Sources of vitamins important in preventing cancer

Vitamin	Sources
A	Vitamin A occurs only in the animal kingdom, and carotenes, from which humans make vitamin A, occur in vegetables. Rich sources are fish liver oils and animal livers. Also in cows milk and egg yolks. Carotenes are in yellow vegetables, parsley and spinach.
B2 (riboflavin)	Yeast, liver, meat, kidneys, milk, all leaf vegetables
B12	Liver, kidneys, meats
C	Green plants, fruits, especially citrus, black currants, berries, tomatoes, capsicums, also found in meats and animal tissues. Vitamin C is destroyed by cooking.
D	Fish liver oils, egg yolk, milk. Formed by the action of sun on the skin.
E	Wheat germ, wholemeal wheat flour

with an increased risk of *stomach cancer, an abnormality of the stomach results in an inability to absorb vitamin B12 from the diet.

Vitamin C: Some studies suggest that a diet chronically low in vitamin C predisposes to cancer of the *stomach and *oesophagus. However, diets low in vitamin C are also low in vitamin A. Vitamin C and vitamin E help to prevent the conversion of nitrates and nitrites to carcinogenic *nitrosamines in the bowel. There is some evidence that **vitamin D** helps prevent *bowel and *breast cancers.

Supplementation of the diet with vitamin pills is not recommended. Vitamins are not all perfectly safe. The water-soluble vitamins are generally safer than the others because, if they are taken in excess, that which is not immediately needed by the body is excreted through the kidneys in the urine. Overdosing with vitamin C can cause deposition of crystals or stones in the bladder and ureters. Prolonged dosing with vitamin C leads to the body adapting to it and disposing of it rapidly. This adaptation lasts for a while after stopping the supplements.

Excessive intake of fat-soluble vitamins can be dangerous. The excess is not so easily excreted, but is stored in body fat. Vitamin A can cause abnormalities of the developing baby in pregnant women. Excess vitamin D can result in serious kidney damage. Overdosage of vitamin E can cause clot formation and high blood pressure.

von Volkmann, Richard 1830–1889, German surgeon who recognized that *tar was the chemical in soot which caused skin cancers. See *chemicals as causes of cancer.

von Recklinghausen's syndrome   described by von Recklinghausen in 1882. Friedrich von Recklinghausen, 1833–1910, was a German pathologist who worked in Strasbourg. See *neurofibromatosis.

VP16–213   trade name of etoposide, medication used in cancer *chemotherapy

W

warning signs of cancer   Everybody should know the common warning signs of cancer. There may be a risk in compiling a list of warning
signs, that persons who tend to be anxious may fear cancer every time
there is a discomfort or minor disturbance. There is only one proper
course if concern arises—see a competent medical practitioner.

Table 20: Symptoms and signs that may warn of cancer

Manifestation	Cancer
1 A sore that does not heal	*skin
2 Change in a wart or a mole	*skin
3 Unusual bleeding or discharge (from bowel, urinary bladder, or any bodily orifice)	*diverse
4 Uterine bleeding after the menopause	*uterus
5 Lumps	*diverse
6 Change in bowel habit	*bowel
7 Cough	*lung
8 Difficulty swallowing	*oesophagus
9 Pain or discomfort	*diverse
10 Hoarseness	*larynx

wart   outgrowth of *cells from the skin, forming a benign tumour,
caused by a *human papilloma virus

water   Various chemical substances are added to domestic water
supplies to make them bacteriologically safe and to improve their
clarity. *Aluminium sulphate is often added during the filtration
process to stick floating organic matter together so that it sinks to the
bottom. Although aluminium is known to have neurotoxic effects and
it has been linked with Alzheimer's disease, the most common form
of dementia, it has not been linked to cancer.

Chlorine, or a blend of chlorine and ammonia, is added to disinfect
the water. *Fluoride is often added to help prevent dental decay, and
*copper sulphate is sometimes added to get rid of algae.

Health problems relating to the addition of chlorine are well
documented. High chlorine concentrations can produce potentially
carcinogenic by-products including *chloroform and other *trihalomethanes. The World Health Organisation (WHO) sets levels of
chloroforms in drinking water which it considers safe.

High levels of chlorine are found after treatment of domestic swimming pools. There seems to be no danger in this, and in any case, the water is not normally ingested.

Drinking water contains *nitrates. Cancer of the stomach has been reported to be more common in certain areas where drinking water has a high nitrate content.

Pollution of seawater is alarming. According to reports, each year more than 11,000 tonnes of heavy *metals reach the North Sea, mainly through rivers, and 11,000 tonnes tonnes of phosphorus and 1.2 million tonnes of nitrous wastes are pumped into the adjacent Baltic Sea. *Polychlorinated biphenyls are only one group of 1000 toxic chemicals identified in dead seals from the North Sea.

To counteract marine pollution, the UK has spent millions of pounds, Denmark has contributed a billion pounds and West Germany has a 5.5 billion pound action plan.

wheat grass   *see alternative cancer treatments

Wilms, M.   1867–1918 German surgeon who became, in succession, professor at Leipzig, Basel and Heidelberg. He described *Wilms' tumour of the kidney in 1899.

Wilms' tumour   type of *kidney cancer. See also *childhood cancer.

Windscale   nuclear power plant in Cumbria, England, now called *Sellafield. On 10 and 11 November 1957, a fire occurred in the plant, leading to the release of radioactive material into the atmosphere, which settled over England, Wales and parts of northern Europe. *Iodine-131 was the most important radioactive substance released. *Polonium-210 and *cesium-137 were also released.

An accidental discharge of radioactive material from the Sellafield reactor was detected by a Greenpeace boat moored off the Cumbrian coast in 1983.

Wittenoom   *asbestos (crocidolite) mine in Western Australia. Up to the end of 1989, 94 of the 6912 men who worked at Wittenoom from 1943 until the mine closed in 1966, had developed *mesothelioma. In addition 20 other cases occurred in contractors and others associated with the mine. On the basis of the long lead time to development of mesothelioma after exposure, it has been predicted that up to 700 more people will develop mesothelioma during the next 30 years. As well as mesothelioma, 141 cases of *lung cancer have occurred and as many more are anticipated. Up to 60% of these will be due to *tobacco and the rest will be attributable to asbestos. See *atomic bombs and nuclear reactors.

wood dust hazard for wood workers, particularly in the furniture industry, associated with cancers of the nasal cavity. See *occupation and cancer.

xeroderma pigmentosum an inherited condition in which cancers occur frequently because of a defective capacity to repair damage to *DNA. See *heredity and cancer, *mutation, *skin cancer.

X-rays short wavelength *electromagnetic radiation, which can cause cancer. Sources of high energy X-rays include diagnostic and therapeutic X-ray machines, *radioactive chemicals, *nuclear reactors and *uranium mines.

Many early radiologists developed cancer and there was a sorry legacy of cancers from medical use in the early days of X-rays. Many conditions other than cancer were treated by X-rays. Cancers of the *bladder, the *thyroid gland in the neck and of the *breast, as well as *leukaemias have been ascribed to this misguided practice. *Ankylosing spondylitis has frequently been treated with X-rays. Subjects so treated are at considerable risk of developing *leukaemia and *multiple myeloma.

Patients receive very small doses from most diagnostic X-ray procedures, equivalent to the annual dose we all receive from cosmic rays. X-rays and radioactive materials have saved far more lives than they have cost. Medical practice would be unthinkable without diagnostic X-rays, and research in cancer (and most branches of medical research) would grind to a halt without the use of radioactive chemicals.

Frequent dental X-rays were once linked to cancer of the *parotid glands. In the early days much greater doses were needed to get X-ray pictures of the teeth than today. During the 1920s, for example, 68 units of radiation (rads) were required to do a full-mouth series of dental X-rays. By 1940 this had dropped to 8.6 units and to only 1.1 units by 1960. Today it is estimated that a dental X-ray series requires only 0.1 of a rad.

The dose of X-rays delivered by modern machines for taking pictures of teeth is therefore quite acceptable if an individual has X-ray examination of teeth every 2 or 3 years over a lifetime.

The unborn child is particularly sensitive to the effects of irradiation and other agents which damage *DNA, with either congenital malformations or cancer as a consequence. The danger of X-rays is greatest in the earliest stages of pregnancy, when the tissues are forming.

Several studies have shown that radiation to the pregnant uterus from diagnostic procedures increases the risk of leukaemia in the child. An Oxford survey of childhood cancer between 1953 and 1979 concluded that about one fatal childhood cancer resulted from every thousand antenatal X-ray examinations. Since then the radiation dose to the unborn child in unavoidable X-ray examinations has halved and the cure rate for childhood leukaemia, the commonest fatal cancer in childhood, has much improved.

The Oxford findings differ from the experience of unborn children of Japanese survivors of the atomic bombs, who were irradiated in the uterus. In the atomic bomb survivors who were born within nine months after the bombing, no increased rate of cancer was seen.

Most of the diagnostic investigation during pregnancy that formerly required X-rays can now be carried out by *ultrasound imaging techniques, which are free from known carcinogenic side-effects. See *medical treatment as a cause of cancer.

Y

Yamagiwa, Katsusaburo 1863–1930, pathologist who studied with *Virchow and became professor in Tokyo. With *Ichikawa he showed in 1911 that repeated painting of *tar on the skin of rabbits would cause *skin cancer. He also showed that other chemicals, for example the dye scarlet red, caused cancer in birds. These observations established that chemical substances could cause cancer. See *chemicals as causes of cancer.

Z

zinc metallic element. Deficiency of zinc may be a causative factor in cancer. See *diet.

Appendix

Sources of Information and Literature for Further Reading

Most of the subjects referred to in this book can be studied in further detail in authoritative textbooks of medicine, such as Harrison's *Principles of Internal Medicine*, or Stein's Internal Medicine, which are available in university and university hospital libraries and can be purchased at university bookshops. Selected references in biomedical journals to recent studies on such subjects as industrial toxins and oral contraceptives are cited.

References in journals are cited here in a standard style of quotation that any librarian can use. The name of the author or authors is followed by the year of publication, then the title of the article, name of the journal, the volume number, and finally first and last pages. The standard abbreviation of the name of the journal is used.

Information on diet and cancer is available from the Dietitians Association of Australia by writing to the Association's executive officer, PO Box 11, O'Connor, ACT, or from any State branch of DAA.

Australian Anti-cancer Foundations

The Australian Cancer Society Inc
GPO Box 4708, SYDNEY, NSW 2001
TELEPHONE (02) 267 1944

ACT Cancer Society
PO Box 509, CANBERRA, ACT 2608
TELEPHONE (062) 48 0726

Anti-Cancer Council of Victoria
1 Rathdowne Street, CARLTON SOUTH, VIC 3053
TELEPHONE (03) 662 3300

Anti-Cancer Foundation of the University of South Australia
PO Box 160, NORTH ADELAIDE, SA 5006
TELEPHONE (08) 267 5222

Cancer Foundation of Western Australia
42 Ord Street, WEST PERTH, WA 6005
TELEPHONE (09) 321 6224

NSW State Cancer Council
GPO Box 7070 SYDNEY, NSW 2001
TELEPHONE (02) 264 8888

Northern Territory Anti-Cancer Foundation
GPO Box 718, DARWIN, NT 5790
TELEPHONE (089) 81 3556

Appendix

Queensland Cancer Fund
PO Box 201, SPRING HILL, QLD 4000
TELEPHONE (07) 839 7077

Tasmanian Cancer Committee
GPO BOX 191B, HOBART, TAS 7001
TELEPHONE (002) 30 6315

Cancer Research

The Clinical Oncology Society of Australia (COSA) provides an annual forum for clinical research on cancer in Australia. While much fundamental laboratory research is reported to other societies, basic research on causation of cancer is also presented to meetings of COSA. COSA also coordinates multicentre clinical trials of cancer treatment and publishes a booklet entitled *Guidelines for the Establishment of Controlled Clinical Trials in Cancer*.

The address of the Clinical Oncology Society of Australia is:

Executive Director, Australian Cancer Society,
GPO BOX 4708, SYDNEY NSW 2001

References

Ades AE, Kazantzis G (1988) Lung cancer in a non-ferrous smelter: the role of cadmium. Br J Ind Med 45:435–442

Barret-Connor E (1989) Postmenopausal estrogen replacement and breast cancer. N Engl J Med 321:319–320

Bannasch P, Editor: *Cancer Risks. Strategies for Elimination* Springer Verlag, Heidelberg, 1987

Berg JW (1976) Nutrition and cancer. Seminars Oncol 3:17–23

Bergkvist L, Adami H-O, Persson I, Hoover R, Schairer C (1989) The risk of breast cancer after estrogen and estrogen-progestin replacement. N Engl J Med 321:293–297

Bertazzi PA, Zocchetti C, Pesatori AC et al. (1989) Ten-year mortality study of the population involved in the Seveso incident in 1976. Am J Epidemiol 129:1187–1200

Bonnett A, Roder D, Esterman A (1989) Epidemiological features of melanoma in South Australia: implications for cancer control. Med J. Aust 151:502–509

Cook-Mozaffari P, Darby S, Doll R (1989) Cancer near potential sites of nuclear installations. Lancet II:1145–1147

Cassel CK, (1989) Chernobyl: learning from experience. N Engl J Med 321:254–255

Chilvers C, Conway D (1985) Cancer mortality in England in relation to levels of naturally occurring fluoride in water supplies. J Epidemiol Community Health 39:44–47

Davis MK, Savitz DA, Graubard BI (1988) Infant feeding and childhood cancer. Lancet II:365–368

Day SB Editor, *Cancer, Stress and Death*, Plenum Publishing Corporation, New York and London, 1986

Eidinger RN, Schapira DV (1984) Cancer patients' insight into their treatment, prognosis and unconventional therapies. Cancer 53:2736–2740

Ekert H, *Childhood Cancer. Understanding and Coping*, Gordon and Breach Science Publishers, New York, London, Paris, Montreux, Tokyo, Melbourne, 1989

Forman D, Cook-Mozaffari P, Darby S et al. (1987) Cancer near nuclear installations. Nature 329:499–505

Gardner MJ, Magnani C, Pannett B, Fletcher AC, Winter PD (1988) Lung cancer among glass fibre production workers: a case-control study. Br J Ind Med 45:613–618

Gaté G *Gabriel Gaté's Family Food*, cookbook commissioned by the Anti-Cancer Council of Victoria, 1987, Penguin Books Aust and NZ

Goldsmith JR (1989) Childhood leukaemia mortality before 1970 among populations near two US nuclear installations. Lancet I:793

Grandjean P, Juel K, Jensen OM (1985) Mortality and cancer morbidity after heavy occupational fluoride exposure. Am J Epidemiol 121:57–64

Hannsen M (1989) *The new additive code breaker*. Lothian Publishing Company Pty Ltd, Melbourne, Sydney, Auckland, 201pp. (This is a reference book to enable the food additive code to the deciphered.)

Hirayama T (1981) Non-smoking wives of heavy smokers have a higher risk of lung cancer: a study from Japan. Br Med J 282:183–185

Järvholm B, Lavenius B (1987) Mortality and cancer morbidity in workers exposed to cutting fluids. Arch Environmental Health 42:361–366

Jones GRN (1989) Polychlorinated biphenyls: where do we stand now? Lancet II:791–794

Kerr RA (1988) Indoor radon: the deadliest pollutant. Science 240:606–608

Keyfitz N (1989 September) The growing human population. Scientific American 261:71–77a. (This article summarises the size and growth of the world's population and analyses effects of the growth. It gives further references.)

Kinlen L (1988) Evidence for an infective cause of childhood leukaemia: comparison of a Scottish new town with nuclear reprocessing sites in Britain. Lancet II: 1323–1327

Kradin RL, Kurnick JT, Lazarus DS et al. (1989) Tumour-infiltrating lymphocytes and interleukin-2 in treatment of advanced cancer. Lancet I:577–580

Appendix

Kübler-Ross, E. (1987) *On Death and Dying*, Tavistock Publications, London.

Lancet Editorial (1988): Antenatal ionizing radiation and cancer. Lancet I:448–449

Lancet Editorial (1988) Life under pylons. Lancet 1:746

Lancet Editorial (1988) Retinoids and the control of cutaneous malignancy. Lancet II:545–546

Lancet Editorial (1989) Adjuvant systemic treatment for breast cancer meta-analysed. Lancet I:80–82

Lancet Editorial (1989) Cancer risks of oral contraception. Lancet I:84

Lancet Editorial (1989) Cancer risks of contraception. Lancet I:21–22

Lancet Editorial (1989) Psychosocial intervention and the natural history of cancer. Lancet II:901

Lancet Leading Article (1990) New treatments for osteoporosis Lancet 335:1065–1066

Lerner IJ (1984) The whys of cancer quackery. Cancer 53 (3 Suppl): 815–819

Lippman SM, Meyskens FL (1987) Treatment of advanced squamous cell carcinoma of the skin with isotretinoin. Ann Int Med 107:499–501

Lucie NP (1989) Radon exposure and leukaemia. Lancet II:99–100

Marx JL (1989) Estrogen use linked to breast cancer. Science 245:593

McMichael AJ (1988) Carcinogenicity of exposure to industrial chemicals. Misconceptions and realities. Medical Toxicology 3:425–429

Modan B, Chetrit A, Alfandary E, Katz L (1989) Increased risk of breast cancer after low-dose irradiation. Lancet I 629–630

Nero AV Jr, (1988, May) Controlling indoor air pollution. Scientific American 258:24–30

Penkett SA (1989) Ultraviolet levels down not up. Nature 341:283–284

Potter JD, McMichael AJ (1986) Diet and cancer of the colon and rectum: a case-control study. J Natl Cancer Inst 76:557–569

Reynolds, P (Trish) (1987) *Your Cancer, Your Life*. Greenhouse Publications, Victoria, Australia 306 pages

Richmond VL (1985) Thirty years of fluoridation: a review. Am J Clin Nutr 41:129–138

Roberts L (1987) Radiation accident grips Goiânia. Science 238:1028–1031

Rosenbaum EH (ed). (1983) *Can you Prevent Cancer? Realistic Guidelines for Developing Cancer — Preventive Life Habits*. CV Mosby Company St Louis, Toronto.

Smigel K (1989) The pill and breast cancer: is there a connection? J Natl Cancer Inst 81:256–257

Smith GH, Williams FL, Lloyd OL (1987) Respiratory cancer and air pollution from iron foundries in a Scottish town: an epidemiological and environmental study. Br J Ind Med 44:795–802

Spiegel D, Bloom JR, Kraemer HC, Gottheil E (1989) Effect of psychosocial treatment on survival of patients with metastatic breast cancer. Lancet II:888–891

Sullivan K, Waterman L (1988) Cadmium and cancer: report of an international meeting in London, September 1988. Ann Occup Hyg 32:557–560

Tattersall M, Editor (1988) *Preventing Cancer*, Australian Professional Publications, Sydney.

Toniolo P, Riboli E, Protta F, Charrel M, Cappa APM (1989) Calorie-providing nutrients and risk of breast cancer. J Natl Cancer Inst 81:278–286

Toxic chemical, radiation and environmental safety. A newsletter (6 issues per year) obtainable from Ecol Data Pty Ltd, PO Box 206, Everton Park, 4053 Queensland

UK Trial of Early Detection of Breast Cancer Group. (1988) First results on mortality reduction in the UK trial of early detection of breast cancer. Lancet II:411–416

Vainio H, Tomatis L, (1985) Exposure to carcinogens: scientific and regulatory aspects. Ann Am Conf Ind Hyg 12:134–143

Vernie LN (1984) Selenium in carcinogenesis. Biochim Biophys Acta 738:203–217

Watson JD, Tooze J *The DNA Story. A Documentary History of Gene Cloning* WH Freeman and Company, San Francisco, 1981

Willett WC, Polk BF, Morris JS et al. (1983) Prediagnostic serum selenium and risk of cancer. Lancet II:130–134

World Health Organisation in collaboration with the Food and Agriculture Organisation of the United Nations: Food irradiation, a technique for preserving and improving the safety of food. Geneva 1988 pp84 ISBN 9241542403

Yoshimoto Y, Kato H, Schull WJ (1988) Risk of cancer among children exposed in utero to A-bomb radiations, 1950–1984. Lancet II:665–669